T0229016

Colonoscopy Quality

Guest Editor

JOHN I. ALLEN, MD, MBA, AGAF

GASTROINTESTINAL ENDOSCOPY CLINICS OF NORTH AMERICA

www.giendo.theclinics.com

Consulting Editor
CHARLES J. LIGHTDALE, MD

October 2010 • Volume 20 • Number 4

SAUNDERS an imprint of ELSEVIER, Inc.

W.B. SAUNDERS COMPANY
A Division of Elsevier Inc.

1600 John F. Kennedy Blvd. • Suite 1800 • Philadelphia, Pennsylvania 19103-2899

http://www.giendo.theclinics.com

GASTROINTESTINAL ENDOSCOPY CLINICS OF NORTH AMERICA Volume 20, Number 4
October 2010 ISSN 1052-5157, ISBN-13: 978-1-4377-2527-8

Editor: Kerry Holland
Developmental Editor: Jessica Demetriou

Gastrointestinal Endoscopy Clinics of North America (ISSN 1052-5157) is published quarterly by Elsevier Inc., 360 Park Avenue South, New York, NY 10010-1710. Months of issue are January, April, July, and October. Business and Editorial Offices: 1600 John F. Kennedy Blvd., Suite 1800, Philadelphia, PA, 19103-2899. Periodicals postage paid at New York, NY and additional mailing offices. Subscription prices are $295.00 per year for US individuals, $414.00 per year for US institutions, $156.00 per year for US students and residents, $325.00 per year for Canadian individuals, $505.00 per year for Canadian institutions, $412.00 per year for international individuals, $505.00 per year for international institutions, and $217.00 per year for Canadian and foreign students/residents. To receive student/resident rate, orders must be accompanied by name of affiliated institution, date of term, and the *signature* of program/residency coordinator on institution letterhead. Orders will be billed at individual rate until proof of status is received. Foreign air speed delivery is included in all *Clinics* subscription prices. All prices are subject to change without notice. **POSTMASTER:** Send address change to *Gastrointestinal Endoscopy Clinics of North America*, Elsevier Health Sciences Division, Subscription Customer Service, 3251 Riverport Lane, Maryland Heights, MO 63043. **Customer Service: 1-800-654-2452 (US). From outside the United States, call 1-314-447-8871. Fax: 1-314-447-8029. E-mail: JournalsCustomerService-usa@elsevier.com (for print support) or JournalsOnlineSupport-usa@elsevier.com (for online support).**

Reprints. For copies of 100 or more, of articles in this publication, please contact the Commercial Reprints Department, Elsevier Inc., 360 Park Avenue South, New York, NY 10010-1710. Tel. (212) 633-3812; Fax: (212) 482-1935; E-mail: reprints@elsevier.com.

Gastrointestinal Endoscopy Clinics of North America is covered in *Excerpta Medica, MEDLINE/PubMed (Index Medicus), and MEDLINE/MEDLARS.*

Printed and bound by CPI Group (UK) Ltd, Croydon, CR0 4YY

Transferred to Digital Print 2011

Contributors

CONSULTING EDITOR

CHARLES J. LIGHTDALE, MD
Professor, Department of Medicine, Columbia University Medical Center, New York, New York

GUEST EDITOR

JOHN I. ALLEN, MD, MBA, AGAF
National Quality Advisor, Minnesota Gastroenterology PA; Clinical Associate Professor of Medicine, University of Minnesota School of Medicine, Minneapolis, Minnesota

AUTHORS

JOHN I. ALLEN, MD, MBA, AGAF
National Quality Advisor, Minnesota Gastroenterology PA; Clinical Associate Professor of Medicine, University of Minnesota School of Medicine, Minneapolis, Minnesota

NIALL J. BRENNAN, MPP
Engelberg Center for Health Care Reform, The Brookings Institution, Washington, DC

ROBERT S. BRESALIER, MD
Professor of Medicine, Resoft Distinguished Professor in GI Oncology, Department of Gastroenterology, Hepatology and Nutrition, The University of Texas M.D. Anderson Cancer Center, Houston, Texas

LAWRENCE B. COHEN, MD
Associate Clinical Professor, Mount Sinai School of Medicine, New York, New York

PIET C. DE GROEN, MD
Consultant, Division of Gastroenterology and Hepatology, Department of Internal Medicine; Division of Biomedical Statistics and Informatics, Department of Health Sciences Research; Professor of Medicine, Mayo Clinic College of Medicine, Rochester, Minnesota

JASON A. DOMINITZ, MD, MHS
Associate Professor, Department of Medicine, Division of Gastroenterology, University of Washington; VA Puget Sound Health Care, Seattle, Washington

DOUGLAS O. FAIGEL, MD
Professor of Medicine, Division of Gastroenterology and Hepatology, Department of Medicine, Oregon Health & Science University, Portland, Oregon

ANDREW D. FELD, MD, JD, FACG, AGAF, FASGE
Clinical Professor, Division of Gastroenterology, University of Washington, Seattle;
Rockwood Clinic; and Group Health Cooperative, Spokane, Washington

KAYLA A. FELD, AB
Harvard University, Cambridge, Massachusetts; Tulane University School of Law; Group
Health Cooperative, Division of Gastroenterology, New Orleans, Louisiana

DAVID GREENWALD, MD
Associate Professor of Clinical Medicine, Albert Einstein College of Medicine; Associate
Division Director of Gastroenterology, Montefiore Medical Center, Bronx, New York

DAVID G. HEWETT, MBBS, FRACP
Division of Gastroenterology, Department of Medicine, Indiana University School
of Medicine, Indianapolis, Indiana; School of Medicine, University of Queensland and
Queensland Health Skills Development Centre, Brisbane, Queensland, Australia

CHARLES J. KAHI, MD, MSc
Division of Gastroenterology, Department of Medicine, Indiana University School
of Medicine, Indianapolis, Indiana

CYNTHIA W. KO, MD, MS
Associate Professor, Department of Medicine, Division of Gastroenterology, University
of Washington, Seattle, Washington

TODD A. LEE, PharmD, PhD
Center for Management of Complex Chronic Care, Hines VA Hospital;
Departments of Pharmacy Practice and Pharmacy Administration, Center for
Pharmacoeconomics Research, University of Illinois at Chicago, Chicago, Illinois

DAVID A. LIEBERMAN, MD
Professor of Medicine and Chief, Division of Gastroenterology and Hepatology,
Department of Medicine, Oregon Health & Science University, Portland, Oregon

JUDITH R. LOGAN, MD
Associate Professor, Department of Medical Informatics and Clinical Epidemiology,
Oregon Health & Science University, Portland, Oregon

CHRISTOPHER S. LYTTLE, MA
Department of Pharmacy Administration, Center for Pharmacoeconomics Research,
University of Illinois at Chicago, Chicago, Illinois

DOUGLAS K. REX, MD
Division of Gastroenterology, Department of Medicine, Indiana University School
of Medicine, Indianapolis, Indiana

DALE C. SNOVER, MD
Department of Pathology, Fairview Southdale Hospital; Clinical Professor
of Laboratory Medicine and Pathology, Edina, Minnesota

KEVIN B. WEISS, MD
Institute for Healthcare Studies, Northwestern University, Chicago, Illinois

ADAM S. WILK, BA
Engelberg Center for Health Care Reform, The Brookings Institution, Washington, DC

JASON E. WILLIAMS, MD, MPH
Gastroenterology Fellow, Division of Gastroenterology and Hepatology, Department of Medicine, Oregon Health & Science University, Portland, Oregon

ANN G. ZAUBER, PhD
Associate Attending, Department of Epidemiology and Biostatistics, Memorial Sloan-Kettering Cancer Center, New York, New York

Contents

> This article reviews potential risk areas and legal issues in quality and colonoscopy. These include issues about open access colonoscopy, informed consent for colonoscopy, missed colorectal cancer, problems related to anticoagulation or its withdrawal for colonoscopy, procedural problems with sedation, failure to follow up appropriately, and failure to identify and warn of high genetic risk.

> Colonoscopy is a well recognized diagnostic and therapeutic tool. Endoscope reprocessing must be done correctly every time; a breach of protocol leading to transmission of infection has the potential to bring endoscopy to a halt. Standards exist that guide the practitioner in all health care settings to minimize the chance of transmission of infection. Safe injection practices and reprocessing of endoscopes using high-level disinfection and sterilization methods may help avert the risk of contracting possible infections during colonoscopy procedures.

> The subject of endoscopic sedation for colonoscopy remains controversial because of unresolved questions concerning the relative benefits, risks, and cost of service. There is also disagreement about the most appropriate sedation drug(s), delegation of responsibility for drug administration, and patient monitoring. This article examines recent trends in endoscopic sedation; the impact of sedation on the quality, safety, and patient tolerability of colonoscopy; and reviews the economic implications of current sedation practices.

> Rapidly evolving knowledge of the pathogenesis and natural history of colorectal cancer (CRC), especially in high-risk groups, is allowing the development of new tools to identify those who will benefit most from

preventive measures. Currently, screening for adenomas, dysplasia, and early-stage invasive cancers provides the best opportunity to prevent and improve survival from CRC. Screening of high-risk groups almost always includes colonoscopy. This review discusses what represents quality colonoscopy. Proper risk stratification, understanding the natural history of each disease, proper patient counseling, and optimal techniques all help define quality colonoscopy in high-risk groups.

Good communication between clinician and pathologist is essential for optimal patient care and management of colorectal polyps and carcinoma. General principles of communication include making sure that the pathologist and endoscopist have all the information needed to make an accurate diagnosis and that the pathologist communicates the diagnosis back to the endoscopist in a clear and timely fashion. The increasing complexity of classification of colorectal polyps and carcinomas has added to the need for clear communication pathways. The first part of this article is devoted to an outline of general communication issues; the second is a discussion of current concepts in colorectal polyps and carcinomas.

Although complications of colonoscopy are rare, they are potentially serious and life threatening. In addition, less serious adverse events may occur frequently and may have an impact on a patient's willingness to undergo future procedures. This article reviews the magnitude of and risk factors for major and minor colonoscopy complications, discusses management of complications, and suggests ways to design quality improvement programs to reduce the risk of complications.

Colonoscopy is sometimes considered the preferred colorectal cancer screening modality, yet this modality may be subject to variation in operator performance more than any other screening test. Failures of colonoscopy to consistently detect precancerous lesions threaten the effectiveness of this technique for the prevention of colorectal cancer. Studies on high-level adenoma detectors under optimal conditions have begun to establish the true efficacy of colonoscopy and further widen the gap between efficacy and effectiveness. Research is required to establish the component skills, attitudes, and behaviors for high-level mucosal inspection competence necessary for training and assessment. Interventions to bridge the gap between efficacy and effectiveness are lacking, yet they should emphasize quality measurement and operate at various levels within the health system to motivate change in endoscopist behavior.

Quality improvement of colonoscopy continues to be an important topic. This effort begins with creating detailed and accurate colonoscopy reports. Quality indicators are measurable endpoints that may be used in quality assurance and improvement plans. Key quality measures include cecal intubation rate, adenoma detection, withdrawal time, preparation quality, follow-up recommendations, and American Society of Anesthesiologists classification. Unresolved issues include establishing proper benchmarks, documenting the correlation between process measures and outcomes, aligning incentives to improved quality outcomes, and issues regarding access to quality data.

Colorectal cancer is the second major cause of cancer-related death in the United States. The long time involved in progression of mucosal dysplasia from a small polyp to an invasive cancer and the ability to image the colon mucosa are features that make early detection and prevention of colorectal cancer by colonoscopy possible. Although colonoscopy has contributed to a marked decline in the number of colorectal cancer-related deaths, the protective effect of colonoscopy, when used in routine clinical practice, has not lived up to the expectations raised by carefully controlled prospective research studies. Therefore new systems that assess quality of colonoscopy are needed.

Administrative databases, registries, and clinical databases are designed for different purposes and therefore have different advantages and disadvantages in providing data for enhancing quality. Administrative databases provide the advantages of size, availability, and generalizability, but are subject to constraints inherent in the coding systems used and from data collection methods optimized for billing. Registries are designed for research and quality reporting but require significant investment from participants for secondary data collection and quality control. Electronic health records contain all of the data needed for quality research and measurement, but that data is too often locked in narrative text and unavailable for analysis. National mandates for electronic health record implementation and functionality will likely change this landscape in the near future.

Working with a group of key stakeholders, the authors developed an episode-based resource use measure focused on the use of colonoscopy. This measure is intended to identify differences in health care resource use in a short time frame surrounding the colonoscopy. The ultimate intent in the development of this measure was to pair it with a measure of quality so that both the cost and quality of care can be evaluated together. In initial testing, the authors found the use of general anesthesia with colonoscopy to be associated with higher episode costs. Eventually, when paired with quality measures, it is hoped this measure will provide actionable information for health care payers and providers to more efficiently provide colonoscopy services without compromising quality.

THE CLINICS ARE NOW AVAILABLE ONLINE!

Access your subscription at:
www.theclinics.com

Foreword

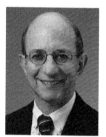

Charles J. Lightdale, MD
Consulting Editor

Colonoscopy for screening, surveillance, and prevention of colorectal cancer is one of the great success stories of modern gastrointestinal endoscopy. In the United States, at least in part because of widespread utilization of colonoscopy, colon cancer incidence and mortality are decreasing. Yet the mass application of colonoscopy in populations at risk has not unexpectedly focused intense scrutiny on colonoscopy practice. For most clinical gastroenterologists, colonoscopy examinations for cancer prevention are a central part of their practice. The electronic medical record and powerful computers will provide rivers of data for analysis of what they actually do and accomplish. How to achieve the highest quality in these procedures at a cost compatible with national health priorities has become a paramount issue.

Probably no one in the country knows more about the critical questions involved with colon cancer screening and colonoscopy practice than John I. Allen, MD, MBA, who is Guest Editor for this issue of *Gastrointestinal Endoscopy Clinics of North America*. Dr Allen is first and foremost not an ivory tower analyst, but rather a practicing gastroenterologist with Minnesota Gastroenterology, St Paul, where he also serves as medical director for quality. Dr Allen, who has extraordinary insights into the practice of gastroenterology in the United States, also holds an appointment at the University of Minnesota, Minneapolis, and has major roles in the American Gastroenterological Association, most recently as chair of the AGA executive management board developing and overseeing a national outcomes registry for gastroenterologists.

When I suggested to Dr Allen that he should be Guest Editor for an issue of *Gastrointestinal Endoscopy Clinics of North America* on the "quality" of colonoscopy, he countered that he preferred to broaden the subject to encompass the "value" of colonoscopy. I accepted immediately, but quickly checked my Oxford English Dictionary for the word "value." The most fitting definition seemed to be: "the relative status of a thing…according to its real worth." How to provide ongoing high value in colonoscopy screening will be a primary concern of practicing gastroenterologists for the foreseeable future. Dr Allen has selected topics authored by the greatest experts

doi:10.1016/j.giec.2010.07.013

and thought leaders in the area. This volume represents an essential guide for practicing gastroenterologists and is a compelling read for all.

Charles J. Lightdale, MD
Department of Medicine
Columbia University Medical Center
161 Fort Washington Avenue, Room 812
New York, NY 10032, USA

E-mail address:
CJL18@columbia.edu

Preface

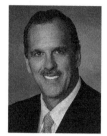

John I. Allen, MD, MBA, AGAF
Guest Editor

A high-quality colonoscopy exam performed by an experienced endoscopist is safe and comfortable and offers patients a high value for their health care dollar. Colonoscopy helps provide accurate assessment of an individual's colorectal cancer (CRC) risk, allows the endoscopist to diagnose prevalent neoplasia, and reduces risk for future CRC when physicians find and remove precancerous polyps. This nation's infrastructure for CRC screening has grown substantially over the last decade and real gains in cancer prevention and survival have been achieved based in part on the effectiveness of colonoscopy. In 2010, colonoscopy is the most widely used CRC screening and surveillance intervention, and approximately 12 million exams are performed annually in the United States. The cost for these exams exceeds $14 billion. It is in the best interest of this nation to maximize the health care value of colonoscopy.

Of all the screening tests endorsed by the United States Preventative Services Task Force, colonoscopy is the most expensive, most invasive, and most dangerous. It also ranks among the most cost effective and clinically effective screening tests for adults. The clinical effectiveness of colonoscopy as a cancer prevention modality relates directly to the quality of the exam. Cost effectiveness of colonoscopy relates to both quality and cost. If quality is substandard or the cost is high, then the health care value is diminished.

The "value" of colonoscopy (or any medical intervention) is defined as Quality/Cost, where quality reflects the Institute of Medicine's (IOM) "Six Aims." The IOM states that medical care should be safe, timely, efficient, effective, equitable, and patient-centered. Cost refers to both the individual cost of an intervention and the overall cost to a population of their medical care. Donald Berwick, MD, past President of the Institute for Healthcare Improvement and now the Director of the Centers for Medicare and Medicaid, has written about the "Triple Aim." Health care should enhance the experience of the individual, increase the health of the nation, and reduce the overall cost of care.

These concepts are important for the endoscopist to understand since there are serious questions concerning results of colonoscopy when used to screen for and prevent CRC. There have been egregious breaks in safety protocols related to both endoscope cleaning and sedation that have resulted in infection transmission from

Gastrointest Endoscopy Clin N Am 20 (2010) xv–xvi
doi:10.1016/j.giec.2010.07.010
1052-5157/10/$ – see front matter © 2010 Elsevier Inc. All rights reserved.

patient to patient. Variations in the cost of colonoscopy are well documented and the rate of CRC diagnosed within 3 years of a "normal" colonoscopy remains a concern.

In this issue, we have tapped the experience and thoughts of many leaders in the field of colonoscopy and CRC prevention. The overall focus of this issue is how we as individual endoscopists, the health care system, and the nation can maximize the health care value of colonoscopy. In the first six articles, the focus is on the individual experience of colonoscopy. Topics include risk management, infection control, sedation issues, management of high-risk individuals, pathology considerations, and procedure complications. The next three articles deal with how we might improve colonoscopy with adequate documentation, performance measures, and advanced imaging and computer analytic technologies. Three articles focus on a national perspective by discussing use of large databases, innovative payment methodologies, and cost-effectiveness analysis. The final article summarizes efforts to maximize the value of colonoscopy in the community setting.

I wish to thank the authors for their valuable contributions and generous donation of their time and intellect. Special thanks goes to Dr Charles Lightdale for seeing the need for this issue and offering me the opportunity to edit. Finally, Kerry Holland and her staff at Elsevier deserve heartfelt thanks for overseeing editing and publication.

John I. Allen, MD, MBA, AGAF
Minnesota Gastroenterology PA
PO Box 14909
Minneapolis, MN 55414, USA

University of Minnesota School of Medicine
420 Delaware Street, SE
Minneapolis, MN 55455, USA

E-mail address:
jallen@mngastro.com

Risk Management and Legal Issues for Colonoscopy

Kayla A. Feld, AB[a,b], Andrew D. Feld, MD, JD, AGAF[c,d,e],*

KEYWORDS

• Colonoscopy • Risk management • Quality • Legal issues

Preventing adverse clinical outcomes for patients and adverse legal actions for legal practice is a laudable goal. The growing interest and body of knowledge supporting quality improvements in colonoscopy hopefully will reduce missed or delayed diagnosis of colon cancer and procedural complications.[1–6] Efforts to ensure quality colonoscopy also may reduce physician liability: if fewer patients experience harm, then fewer cases will result in litigation. The quality movement, however, can be a double-edged legal sword. As quality measures and processes become established, they may become de facto standards of care, and thus physician noncompliance with reputable quality measures and guidelines may be construed as failure to provide standard of care with adverse effects during a malpractice trial. Given the increasingly public nature of quality measures and professional and society interest in improving quality, it will not be possible to ignore quality measures without increasing litigation exposure.[5] The careful gastroenterologist will need to keep up with quality issues and measures both for good patient care and for risk management.

This article reviews some potential risk areas in quality and colonoscopy. These include issues about open-access colonoscopy, informed consent for colonoscopy,[7] missed colorectal cancer (CRC) (delayed diagnosis in legal parlance),[8] problems

---

The information in this article is presented for general information purposes, and should not be construed to provide specific legal advice to individuals; that would require consultation with an attorney.

[a] Harvard University, Massachusetts Hall Cambridge, MA 02138, USA
[b] Tulane University School of Law, 6329 Freret Street, New Orleans, LA 70118, USA
[c] University of Washington, Division of Gastroenterology, 1959 NE Pacific Street, PO Box 356424, Seattle, WA 98195-6424, USA
[d] Rockwood Clinic, Division of Gastroenterology, 400 East 5th Avenue, Spokane, WA 99202, USA
[e] Group Health Cooperative, Division of Gastroenterology, 125 16th Avenue East, CSB-2, Seattle, WA 98112, USA
* Corresponding author. Rockwood Clinic, Division of Gastroenterology, 400 East 5th Avenue, Spokane, WA 99202.
E-mail address: afeld@uw.edu

Gastrointest Endoscopy Clin N Am 20 (2010) 593–601
doi:10.1016/j.giec.2010.07.002
1052-5157/10/$ – see front matter © 2010 Elsevier Inc. All rights reserved.

related to anticoagulation or its withdrawal for colonoscopy, procedural problems with sedation,[9] failure to follow up appropriately, and failure to identify and warn of high genetic risk.[10,11]

RISK MANAGEMENT

A risk management program is intended to mitigate legal risk through prevention and implementation of proactive strategies. These programs involve estimation of actual risk by analysis of malpractice data so that a risk reduction strategy can be developed based on empiric data. Exact data are frequently difficult to find, so physicians should understand the concept of reasonable risk, based on legal theory. For instance, realizing that physicians have a duty to warn patients and families with high genetic risk of CRC will lead them to develop policies to ensure appropriate patient warnings.[12] Such programs endeavor to clarify areas where legal risk occurs, and introduce strategies to anticipate and manage risk without contributing unduly to costly defensive medicine, in which alternative modes of medical practice are used principally to forestall possibility litigation rather than to provide quality care.[13]

An actuarial assessment of malpractice risk[14] has revealed that delayed diagnosis of CRC is the most frequent and serious lawsuit against gastroenterologists. Understanding tort of negligence, the basis for most medical malpractice suits, will explain why these are attractive cases for a plaintiffs attorney.[15] Plaintiff attorneys must prove four elements:

1. The physician has an obligation (duty) of care for the individual
2. The duty was violated (breach) by practice below applicable standards of care
3. That substandard practice caused the harm asserted (proximate cause)
4. The plaintiff suffered compensable damages (harm).

CRC is a serious illness that produces significant harm, which can be associated with a large financial damages award. The potential for a large financial settlement or court judgment is enough to justify the expense a malpractice plaintiff's attorney will front to bring a lawsuit forward. If the attorney believes the critical elements of a negligence claim can be met, particularly a breach of standard of care or informed consent, a colon cancer claim will likely be pursued. However, if the careful gastroenterologist has practiced within the standard of care and with appropriate informed consent, then despite the patient's damages, the plaintiff's attorney must be concerned a jury will decide the problem was a bad outcome and not medical negligence. In that situation, it is risky for the plaintiff's attorney to take a contingency fee case in which the law firm may lose substantial money spent on expert witnesses, depositions, court fees, and the like. A gastroenterologist practicing within established quality measures is a harder malpractice target.

Thus a review of potential problems of standard of care and informed consent arising from quality aspects of colonoscopy may be helpful in ensuring one's policies and practice meet evolving standards of care. Adopting quality standards is likely to benefit patients, help marketing and business efforts, and benefit the practitioner in the event of legal malpractice challenge.

Ignoring quality standards is realistically not an option. Sufficient data exist about practices that a plaintiff's attorney can often build a case against those who elect not to measure quality. For instance, a malpractice claim was made against a gastroenterologist who used photo documentation during colonoscopy. The view of the cecum was timed, as was the retroflexed rectal view, which occurred 1 minute after the cecal view. It is easier for an attorney to prove substandard colonoscopy technique when a gastroenterologist fails consistently to monitor recommended quality standards.

SPECIFIC ISSUES IN RISK MANAGEMENT FOR QUALITY COLONOSCOPY
Clinical Guidelines

Establishing that a provider violated the standard of care is often the most critical element of a lawsuit. Expert witness testimony is required to establish current standards of care. With increasing frequency, respected national guidelines are relied upon in the event of a lawsuit to define standards of care: that which a reasonable and prudent member of the medical profession would undertake under the same or similar circumstances.[16,17] The plaintiff's attorney often will use these recommendations to determine if the physician has provided that standard of care and to decide whether to take a malpractice case. Clinical guidelines also are used to supplement and enhance expert testimony. Clinical guidelines frequently are used to define standard of care, even if guidelines state they have been developed to enhance clinical care and not for legal purposes.[17] Legal scholars predict this trend will become even stronger.[18]

Quality measures are based on recommendations provided by large organizations with expertise in the area described. For colonoscopy, groups such as the American College of Gastroenterology, the American Gastroenterology Association, and the American Society for Gastrointestinal Endoscopy would provide evidence and consensus-based standards for improving overall quality of gastrointestinal (GI) procedures[1,3,4] and reducing the variability of performance. Documents by societies of that stature likely would influence expert witness testimony and be convincing to a jury charged with assessing appropriate standards of care.

Quality measures may appear on the surface different than clinical guidelines. However, expert witnesses may cite quality measures in the same manner as clinical guidelines. Little imagination is required to understand how a jury could be persuaded that quality measures should be regarded as standards of care. Influential texts such as "To Err is Human: Building a Safer Health System"[19] and "Crossing The Quality Chasm: A New Health System For The 21st Century"[20] have only heightened public concern about medical error and the quality of medical care. Medical societies are responding with a multitude of programs, task forces, and quality measures to help achieve clinical quality.[1,3,4] It will be increasingly necessary for the practicing gastroenterologist to be aware of those measures, and adopt those that are likely to be construed as standard of care, or face challenges in the event of a negligence claim. While these measurements may theoretically put a physician at risk by showing the physician conducted a low-quality examination, they will more often play a useful role in demonstrating that the physician did comply with accepted standard of care. As previously noted, if physicians do not track accepted quality standards, some outcomes may be inferred from photo documentation or records review. A court might instruct physicians who do not track adenoma detection rates to comply with a discovery request from the plaintiff's attorney for that rate by going through records and calculating it retrospectively. The difficulty of such a process would not necessarily dissuade the court, which places a high premium on accurate discovery.

Open-Access Colonoscopy

Open access (OA) has become well established in gastroenterology. It fulfills multiple business and medical goals, including patient convenience, cost reduction, ease of access, meeting patient/provider request (ie, accomplishing screening colonoscopy in a single visit). Additionally, it is financially rewarding for practices. It is an important part of meeting public health goals in CRC screening. OA has been widely accepted, is widely practiced, and thus is considered to fall within standard of care for gastroenterology.

However, departure from the traditional consultation approach does raise certain potential problems regarding patient/provider expectations, adequate preprocedure screening for indications and safety, informed consent and vicarious liability, and follow-up. In particular, patients too ill to safely undergo the procedure or those who require special attention as a result of anticoagulation or sedation issues may present a problem for the proceduralist who is unaware of those issues or becomes aware only at the last moment. Preprocedural screening is necessary to evaluate whether the patient is healthy enough to undergo the examination and whether any special precautions need be addressed. OA is not a free pass to ignore issues that would have been dealt with in a preprocedural consultation. One should assume that legal challenges might be presented if there were problems with a procedure performed in an OA system and the patient was too ill, or otherwise inappropriate, especially if this information could have been detected with prior consultation. The gastroenterologist could not convincingly shift blame to the referring physician for inadequately supplied information. Preprocedure screening in the OA milieu must be sufficient to prevent inappropriate examinations.

Preprocedure information needed in an OA system should include a sufficient medical history of advanced pulmonary or cardiac disease, allergies, medications (chronic narcotic and anxiolytics), presence of internal devices that might complicate the procedure (eg, automatic cardiac implantable defibrillators, pacemakers, cardiac stents, home oxygen, and continuous positive airway pressure machines). Appropriate decisions can be made during remote or telephone triage regarding the need for bridging anticoagulation or use of anesthesiologists, procedure performance in a hospital facility, or other deviations from normal procedure.

Informed consent and patient expectations are also important issues to manage when considering OA. Special attention is needed to convey adequate information ahead of the procedure, allowing the patient sufficient time to ask questions, and to reduce risks of a challenge based on last-minute or coerced consent.[7] This is particularly true where there are additional risks, such as in anticoagulated or difficult to sedate patients, or for anxious patients with procedural concerns.

Informed Consent

The ethical and legal requirement to obtain informed consent before performing colonoscopy derives from the concept of personal (patient) autonomy.[21] The competent patient, after receiving appropriate disclosure of the material risks of the procedure, understanding those risks, the benefits, and the alternative approaches, makes a voluntary and uncoerced informed decision to proceed.[22] A physician violates his or her duty to this patient and subjects himself or herself to liability when any facts necessary to form the basis of intelligent consent by the patient to proposed treatment are withheld.[23]

Malpractice suits using the doctrine of informed consent generally rely upon one of two causes of action:

1. The provision of treatment without obtaining prior consent
2. The failure to disclose sufficient information that would allow for the patient to make a truly informed decision.[24]

Because the latter is more easily proven, cases involving incomplete disclosure are more commonly argued.

The physician has a legal and professional obligation to obtain consent from the patient. This duty serves as more than a procedural requirement to obtain a signature, but rather constitutes a comprehensive process that allows the physician and the patient to achieve a mutual understanding of the risks, alternatives, and goals of the proposed treatment. The physician must ensure that the patient is capable of making an informed and voluntary decision about whether to undergo the proposed treatment. This includes an understanding of the possible material risks associated with the procedure and the availability of alternate treatment options. Material risks[25] are determined by the nature, magnitude, probability, and imminence of the risk that they represent.

Courts apply two different standards to determine the physician's obligation to disclose certain information to a patient: the reasonable person standard and the prudent physician standard. The former requires that physicians disclose what a reasonable person would find significant in deciding about a treatment. Under the prudent physician approach, the information disclosed must comply with that which a reasonable physician in similar circumstances would disclose. Which standard applies depends upon the state in which the gastroenterologist practices.

The process of obtaining informed consent is both a basic ethical obligation and also a legal requirement for physicians. Rather than viewing this process as yet another bureaucratic detail, the informed consent procedure should be viewed as constructive and beneficial for both parties. It allows the patient to gain an understanding of the proposed treatment and the risks involved, as well as learn about alternatives or voice any concerns or questions. The physician has the opportunity to ask about the patient's treatment goals and discover any patient-specific information that will enable the most optimal choice of treatment.

Most state laws specify that obtaining informed consent is a nondelegable duty (ie, it must be performed by the physician and cannot be relegated to ones staff or endoscopy nurse). However, consent is a process, and if sufficient and thorough information is provided, the final portion, in which the physician finalizes consent before the procedure and asks if there any questions remaining, may be very brief. This is most important for the success of an OA process, so that OA patients have already received information, and have been given the opportunity to ask questions to satisfaction, before the preparation for the procedure. The thoroughness of the information packet or process can make it hard to convince a jury that the patient received insufficient information or was coerced even if the final immediate preprocedure discussion with the physician was limited.[7]

A risk management recommendation relevant for OA informed consent includes an intake/preparation process in which the patient is mailed or verbally given information about the procedure. This would cover the purpose, description of the procedure, risks, benefits, and alternatives. It would be useful to instruct and document the patient's receipt of information and if any concerns or questions occur after having read it. Further, one could instruct office staff to be alert to patients who appear uncertain, have many questions, or are worried about proceeding and have staff arrange a preprocedure consultation. On the day of procedure, the physician can fulfill his or her legal obligation by summarizing the information. One possible example: "The information you received noted that no test is perfect, including this endoscopy, and our staff have reviewed the risks of colonoscopy, including bleeding, perforation, infection, heart or respiratory complications, missed diagnosis, incomplete procedure, and sedation risks. Do you have any questions for me?"

Missed Colon Cancer

An interval CRC is traditionally defined as one that occurs within 3 years of a negative colonoscopy. This situation carries significant liability risk for the gastroenterologist, and is devastating for the patient and his or her family. The legal issue hinges on whether the standard of care during performance of the colonoscopy was breached. Two questions are central to final legal resolution. First, was the cancer newly developed since the examination because it was fast growing? Second, was the procedure performed with good technical quality, defined as a level of talent that a reasonable physician in similar circumstances would have applied? The later implies that the average gastroenterologist would not have detected the cancer at first colonoscopy.

The general public usually does not realize that even the most careful endoscopist cannot guarantee a 100% detection rate of CRC. Even a physician recognized to be highly skilled still may face legal action if he or she fails to understand and document using protocols recommended by medical literature. A list of generally acceptable components of complete documentation for colonoscopy includes the following

Photographic recording of the cecum
Description of the colon preparation (with a recommendation for early repeat when the prep is inadequate
Slow and careful withdrawal with adequate clearing of residual pools of liquid
Compliance with informed consent process, including mention of missed diagnosis
An established process for managing postprocedure patient inquiries or complications
A secure method to notify patients and referring physicians of procedure results (including pathology and including recommendations for further examinations)
Some system to monitor procedure quality and results.[8]

Anticoagulation

Patients taking anticoagulant medication require additional consideration by the physician. In some instances, temporarily taking the patient off medication may prove necessary to prevent internal bleeding during or after the procedure. However, one must weigh the risks of thrombosis or cardiac stent occlusion with risks caused by discontinuing anticoagulation or antiplatelet therapy. These risks must be explained to the patient and his or her consent documented. Treating physicians have been found liable in a wrongful death suit where the patient was instructed to stop anticoagulant medication for what was concluded to be an excessive period of time.[26]

Sedation

The physician's duty to identify and manage medical circumstances that require special attention applies directly to issues concerning sedation (see the article by Cohen elsewhere in this issue). Physicians should identify prior sedation issues, a medical status that could complicate sedation (eg, emphysema, cardiomyopathy, obstructive sleep apnea, use of home oxygen or continuous positive airway pressure [CPAP]) and medications that might render certain sedatives ineffective (chronic narcotics and anxiolytics). For patients with increased risk, physicians might elect to perform the procedure within a hospital setting and consider having an anesthesiologist administer sedation. Failure to document whether these issues were considered and managed in a generally acceptable manner could result in liability for negligence.[9]

Failure to Follow Up

A physician's duty to his or her patients extends to post-treatment follow-up. The physician should inform the patient of polyp histology and recommend follow-up care that complies with professional guidelines as published in the medical literature.

Failure to recommend appropriate follow-up care has resulted in physicians being found negligent.[27] Clinical guidelines from GI societies are especially relevant in this situation. Further, mistakes made by office personnel who fail to communicate physician-directed information may leave the physician liable under the legal theory of vicarious liability (the wrong doing is extended to the person in whose behalf the wrongdoer acted).[15] A process by which future notification of the patient for follow-up examinations should be established within a practice policy manual, and patients must be informed of the importance of follow-up examinations (including the risks of ignoring advise) plus the extent to which the practice will go to find the patient when a follow-up examination is due. The responsibility for notification should be clear to the patient, specialist, and primary care physician.

Genetic Risk

Progress in the field of genetics has opened new possibilities in medical practice and liability. Physicians should understand that certain high-risk genetic conditions give rise to a duty to warn patients, and inform patients of their need to warn family members of the health risks that arise from a possible inherited CRC risk. Although physicians traditionally do not have a duty to third parties (family members who have not established care with the physician) with regards to conditions such as a Lynch syndrome, hereditary nonpolyposis colorectal cancer, and familial adenomatous polyposis (FAP), courts have found physicians at fault for not documenting a clear explanation about the condition and the need for a patient to warn his or her relatives of a potential inherited risk.[10,12]

The most serious concern for the colonoscopist results from a failure to obtain (and document) sufficient family history for a reasonable provider to identify a familial risk. This can be difficult in an OA setting. A plaintiff's attorney may argue the patient presented for CRC risk reduction (which includes both screening and management of future risk), not merely a single colonoscopy. Thus, when a genetic risk is not recognized and managed, this could be construed as negligence. An intake process for OA patients that will identify potential genetic risk may mitigate legal risk and help patients and their families make informed health decisions.

RISK MANAGEMENT PROGRAM

Given the quality issues discussed, an example of a risk management program can be presented. Elements of a risk management program regarding quality colonoscopy may include a codified peer review process, unit reviews, and methods to update as new information becomes available.[28] Certain information, such as complication rates and discussions, should be identified as covered within a formal peer review process, so that mandatory disclosure is limited. However, groups may choose to make some practice (or even physician)-level data public to highlight their concern and openness regarding quality issues. Unless discoverable data show persistently uncorrected substandard performance, openness should not put the physician at increased liability risk. Indeed, it may reflect self-confidence, concern for quality, and acceptable quality performance.

An example of a quality improvement program that provides acceptable risk management might include the following elements

A formal peer review process, which may include reviews of complications, cecal intubation rates, polyp or adenoma detection rates, and colon withdrawal times
Unit review processes, with monitoring of infection control steps (see the article by Greenwood elsewhere in this issue), life support equipment, staff training,

adequacy of colon preparations, adequacy of the reminder systems, results notification with documented follow-up recommendations, adequacy of clinical triage for OA, documentation of sedation recovery, a check-list for discharge instructions, a written policy for responding to postprocedure patient concerns or complications, and sentinel event review

Additional factors: the use of guidelines and plans surrounding anticoagulation and sedation risks; processes for consent, disclosure, and decision making; and methods to obtain family history and manage high-risk conditions as discussed previously

Methods to update both physician and unit reviews as new information becomes available.

Patient registries have become a useful and important epidemiologic tool for learning about quality issues, and especially those requiring numerically large samples. Many contain deidentified data. The legal risk of contributing to a registry is low if the registry has acceptable processes for deidentifying critical patient information and is compliant with the 1996 Health Insurance Portability and Accountability Act (HIPAA). Information needed for malpractice discovery would be obtained by disclosure requests made directly to the gastroenterologist's office and not to a formal registry.

SUMMARY

The overarching aim of quality measurement and improvement with regards to performance of colonoscopy is to enhance the health value of the examination by reducing the risk of missed cancers, avoiding delays in diagnosis or treatment, and minimizing procedural complications. When practiced according to generally acceptable norms, a physician's risk management program should reduce physician liability. As quality measures and processes have become established, they are now being considered factors that define a community standard of care. Thus, physician noncompliance with reputable quality measures and guidelines may be construed as failure to provide standard of care and may affect the result of a malpractice trial. Given the increasingly public nature of quality measures, plus professional and society interest in enhancing the value of colonoscopy, it will be difficult to ignore quality measures. The careful gastroenterologist must keep abreast of changes in quality issues and measures both for good patient care and for risk management.

REFERENCES

1. Brotman M, Allen JI, Bickston SJ, et al. AGA Task Force on quality in practice: a national overview and implications for GI practice. Gastroenterology 2005; 129(1):361–9.
2. Lieberman DA. A call to action-measuring the quality of colonoscopy. N Engl J Med 2006;355:2588–9.
3. Rex DK, Bond JA, Winawer S, et al. Quality in the technical performance of colonoscopy and the continuous quality improvement process for colonoscopy: recommendations for the US multisystem task force on colorectal cancer. Am J Gastroenterol 2002;97:1296–308.
4. Lieberman DA, Nadel M, Smith RA, et al. Standardized colonoscopy reporting and data system report of the Quality Assurance Task Group on the National Colorectal Cancer Round Table. Gastrointest Endosc 2007;65:757–66.

5. Allen JI, Brill JV. Finally, endoscopy quality measures become a reality. AGA Perspectives 2008;4:8–9.
6. Faigel DO, Pike IM, Baron TH, et al. Quality indicators for gastrointestinal endoscopic procedures. Gastrointest Endosc 2006;63:S1–38.
7. Feld AD. Informed consent for colonoscopy. In: Waye J, Rex DK, Williams CB, editors. Colonoscopy: principles and practice. Malden (MA): Blackwell Publishing; 2009. p. 79–89.
8. Rex DK, Bond JH, Feld AD. Medical legal risks of incident cancers after clearing colonoscopy. Am J Gastroenterol 2001;96(4):952–7.
9. Cohen LB, DeLegge M, Aisenberg J, et al. AGA institute review of endoscopic sedation. Gastroenterology 2007;133:675–701.
10. Feld AD. Medicolegal implications of colon cancer screening. Gastrointest Endosc Clin N Am 2002;12(1):171–9.
11. Feld AD. Malpractice risks associated with colon cancer and inflammatory bowel disease. Am J Gastroenterol 2004;9:1641–4.
12. Safer v Pack, 677 A2d 1188, cert. Den'd, 683 A2d1163 (New Jersey 1996).
13. Pengalis SE, Wachsman HF. American law of medical malpractice. 2nd edition. 1992. p. 49.
14. Gerstnberger PD, Plumeri PL. Malpractice claims in gastrointestinal endoscopy: analysis of an insurance industry database. Gastrointest Endosc 1993;39:132–8.
15. Feld AD, Moses RE. Most doctors win: what to do if sued for malpractice. Am J Gastroenterol 2009;6:1346–51.
16. Hood v Phillips 554SW2d 160, 165 (Texas 1977).
17. Moses RE, Feld AD. Legal risks of clinical practice guidelines. Am J Gastroenterol 2008;103:7–11.
18. Mello MM. Of swords and shields: the role of clinical practice guidelines in medical malpractice ligation. Univ PA Law Rev 2001;149(3):645–710.
19. Kohn LT, Corrigan JM, Donaldson MS, editors. To err is human: building a safer health system. Washington, DC: National Academy Press; 2000.
20. Crossing the quality chasm. A new health system for the 21st century. Washington, DC: National Academy Press; 2000.
21. Schleondorff v Society of New York Hospital, 211 N.Y.125, 105 N.E. 92 (1914), New York.
22. Berg JW, Appelbaum PS, Lidz CW, et al. Informed consent: legal theory and clinical practice. 2nd edition. Oxford: Oxford University Press; 2001.
23. Salgo v Leland Stanford Jr. University Board of Trustees 317 P.2d 170, California.
24. Gatter R. Informed consent law and the forgotten duty of physician inquiry. Loyola Univ Chicago Law J 2000;31:557.
25. Canterbury v Spence 464 F.2d 772(D.C. Cir) Washington, DC; 1972.
26. Mitchell v United States, 141 F3d 8; 49 (1st Cir 1998).
27. Bosco v Janowitz, 388 Ill.App.3d 450, 451–2 (2009), Illinois.
28. Petrini DA, Petrini JL. Risk assessment and management for endoscopists in an ambulatory surgery center. Gastrointest Endosc Clin N Am 2006;16:801–15.

Reducing Infection Risk in Colonoscopy

David Greenwald, MD[a,b],*

KEYWORDS

• Infection • Endoscopy • Disinfection • Reprocessing

Maximizing the value of colonoscopy begins with assuring that the procedure is as safe as possible. In the United States alone, more than 10 million colonoscopic procedures are estimated to be performed annually.[1] Colonoscopy is a well-recognized diagnostic and therapeutic tool; complications are rare. Maintenance of effective infection-control processes is a key component of safety, and proper reprocessing of endoscopic equipment is a critical part of any procedure. Meticulous attention to detail during the reprocessing of flexible endoscopic instruments is crucial. Effective cleaning and disinfection of the endoscope is an integral part of the procedure.

Endoscope reprocessing must be done correctly every time; a breach of protocol leading to transmission of infection has the potential to bring the field of endoscopy to a halt. Standards concerning infection control in endoscopy have been developed and disseminated widely since the late 1980s, helping to ensure continued safety in gastrointestinal (GI) endoscopy.[2,3] Physicians and associates working in settings where colonoscopy is performed need to be vigilant about strict adherence to all infection-control and reprocessing guidelines.

POTENTIAL INFECTION RISKS DURING COLONOSCOPY

Standards exist that guide the practitioners in all health care settings to minimizing the chance of transmission of infection. The potential for transmitting infection during colonoscopy exists when there is a breakdown in adherence to such standards. In general, the key issues in reducing the risk of transmission of infection during colonoscopy center on adhering to "best practices" in terms of:

1. General infection-control principles
2. Safe injection practices
3. Endoscope reprocessing.

No financial support.
The author has nothing to disclose
[a] Albert Einstein College of Medicine, 1300 Morris Park Avenue, Bronx, NY 10461, USA
[b] Division of Gastroenterology, Montefiore Medical Center, 111 East 210th Street, Bronx, NY 10467, USA
* Division of Gastroenterology, Montefiore Medical Center, 111 East 210th Street, Bronx, NY 10467.
E-mail address: dgreenwa@montefiore.org

Gastrointest Endoscopy Clin N Am 20 (2010) 603–614
doi:10.1016/j.giec.2010.07.001
1052-5157/10/$ – see front matter © 2010 Elsevier Inc. All rights reserved.

General Infection-Control Principles

Recommended practices for the prevention of transmission of infection in health care settings are available in guidelines that have been promulgated and widely disseminated. The latest Centers for Disease Control and Prevention (CDC) guidelines were published in 2007, and is a comprehensive review that should be part of the standard operating practices for any facility where colonoscopy is performed.[4]

Personal protective equipment such as gowns, gloves, eye protection, and respiratory protective devices should be easily available and used regularly as appropriate to protect endoscopy personnel from exposure to blood, chemicals, and other potentially hazardous materials.

Both the CDC and the Occupational Safety and Health Administration (OSHA) require the use of gloves when touching blood or other potentially infectious materials.[4,5] The CDC recommends the use of masks and eye protection (or a face shield) during patient care activities that are "likely to generate splashes or sprays of blood, body fluids, secretions and excretions." OSHA recommends the use of such equipment whenever "splashes, spray, splatter or droplets of other infectious materials may be generated and eye, nose or mouth contamination can be reasonably anticipated." Thus, recommendations for the use of eye protection and a mask or a face shield allow some discretion and may be subject to interpretation. Both CDC and OSHA recommend the use of protective aprons or gowns when appropriate.[4,5]

Hand washing should occur after contact with any potentially infectious or contaminated items. The CDC recommends that hands should be washed immediately after gloves are removed, after contact between patients, and in some situations, during examination of the same patient to prevent cross-contamination of different sites.

Safe Injection Practices

Safe injection practices are part of high-quality medical care in all settings, including sites where colonoscopy is performed. Several outbreaks of hepatitis C virus infection have occurred in endoscopy centers, ultimately traced to improper injection practices. Improper use of single and multidose anesthetic vials, reuse of needles and syringes, and improper use of intravenous tubing and connectors have all been implicated for spreading infection. In a well-publicized case in Las Vegas, Nevada, in 2008, at least 6 people developed acute hepatitis C. In this situation, cross-contamination between patients occurred after syringes that were reused to draw additional doses of anesthetic from single-use vials were then subsequently used for other patients undergoing endoscopy.[6] CDC guidelines relevant to safe injection practices during endoscopy include the following[4]:

- Use aseptic technique
- Do not administer medications from a syringe to multiple patients, even if the needle or the cannula on the syringe is changed
- Use fluid infusion sets for one patient only
- Use single-dose vials whenever possible
- Do not administer medications from single-dose vials to multiple patients
- If multidose vials must be used, both the needle or cannula and syringe used to access the multidose vial must be sterile
- Do not keep multidose vials in immediate patient treatment areas.

The need to maintain safe injection practices and be vigilant over the injection practices of all staff working in endoscopy cannot be overemphasized.

Endoscope Reprocessing

Guidelines for reprocessing endoscopes, when followed meticulously, prevent any transmission of infection from one patient to the next. Similarly, reprocessing guidelines for other items used during GI endoscopy (accessories, general medical equipment) are specified by the manufacturer and must be followed meticulously. All items used in GI endoscopy must be reprocessed according to guidelines and manufacturer's instructions to prevent cross-contamination.[7,8]

MECHANISM OF TRANSMISSION AND LEVEL OF RISK

Transmission of infection at the time of GI endoscopy is exceedingly rare. When reviewed critically, most cases of infection deemed related to an endoscopic procedure can be traced to the failure to adhere to published guidelines for reprocessing.[8–11] Mechanisms of transmission can be further divided into these broad areas:

1. Procedural errors in the meticulous cleaning and disinfection of the endoscope, leading to retained microorganisms on the endoscope. These organisms may accumulate in the crevices and joints of the instruments.
2. Insufficient exposure time to liquid chemical germicides (LCGs) or use of inappropriate disinfectant solutions.
3. Improper use of automated endoscope reprocessing equipment.
4. Contaminated water bottles and irrigating solutions.
5. Inadequate drying and improper storage of endoscopes after reprocessing.

The reported frequency of transmission of infection in GI endoscopy has been estimated to be 1 in 1.8 million.[11] This much-quoted rate emanates from Spach and colleagues[12] in 1993, who reviewed 281 infections related to GI endoscopy, as well as 96 thought to have been caused by bronchoscopy (**Table 1**). Of the 281, all but 28 occurred before 1988, the year when importance of adequate manual cleaning as well as disinfection were stressed in guidelines published by the American Society for Gastrointestinal Endoscopy (ASGE) and the British Society of Gastroenterology (BSG).[13,14] The ASGE Technology Committee reviewed Spach's data in 1993 and then estimated that 40 million GI procedures had been done in the United States between 1988 and 1992. This meant there had been 28 reported infections in approximately 40 million endoscopic procedures, for an estimated rate of transmission of infection by GI endoscopy of 1 in 1.8 million. Some think that with widespread adoption of the Multi-Society Guidelines in 2003 the actual transmission rate of infection via endoscopy is considerably lower, with estimates in the 1 in 6 million range.[15]

However, it is also possible that the reported infection rate is underestimated because of factors such as inadequate surveillance, asymptomatic infections, and infections with long incubation periods.[16,17] Some investigators have suggested that endoscopists do not capture all their complications because follow-up is too short; infectious complications might not be recognized to be related to the procedure, or the patient may return to another caregiver or facility and the complication is never apparent to the health care provider who completed the procedure. These investigators recommended a 30-day follow-up of GI procedures (as opposed to the traditional assessment of complications recognized during and immediately after the procedure) as a better measure to study endoscopic complications.[18]

Every patient must be considered as a potential source of infection, and all endoscopes must be reprocessed in a standardized fashion. It is crucial to understand that all recent cases of pathogen transmission related to endoscopy have been the

Table 1
Microorganisms transmitted by (or shown to contaminate) endoscopes: major factors involved in incident (indicated by X)

	Infection (I) or Contamination (C)	Cleaning Procedure	Disinfection Process	Rinsing Process	Automated Processor	Contaminated Processing or Water Bottle
Before Guidelines						
A. Gram-negative bacilli						
Pseudomonas aeruginosa	I	X	X	X	X	X
Klebsiella sp	I	X	X			
Enterobacter sp	I	X	X			
Serratia marcescens	I	X	X			
Salmonella sp including S typhi	I	X	X			X
Helicobacter pylori	I	X	X			X
Bacillus sp	C	X	X			
Proteus sp	C	X	X			
B. Mycobacteria						
Mycobacterium tuberculosis	I	X	X			
Atypical mycobacteria	I	X	X			
C. Fungi						
Trichosporon sp	C		X		X	X

Rhodotorula rubra	C	X	X	X
D. Parasites				
Strongyloides	I	X	X	
E. Viruses				
Hepatitis B	I	X	X	
After Guidelines				
A. Gram-negative bacilli				
P aeruginosa	I	X	X	
B. Mycobacteria				
M tuberculosis	I	X	X	X
Atypical mycobacteria	C	X	X	
C. Viruses				
Hepatitis C	I	X	X	X

Data from Alvarado CJ, Reichelderfer M. APIC guidelines for infection prevention and control in flexible endoscopy. Am J Infect Control 2000;28:138–55.

result of a breach in following accepted protocols. Reprocessing standards are published, updated, and widely available, and include the Multi-Society Guidelines (2003), as well as individual guidelines from the ASGE (2008), Society for Gastrointestinal Nurses and Associates (SGNA) (2008), European Society for Gastrointestinal Endoscopy (2008), Association of Perioperative Registered Nurses (AORN) (2002), and BSG (1998).[2,3,19–22]

SPECIFIC STEPS AND METHODS TO REDUCE INFECTION RISK IN THE ENDOSCOPY UNIT

Adherence to standardized methodology is the most important step in reducing or eliminating the risk of infection transmission in GI endoscopy. Reprocessing is a crucial step in the entire procedure; proper attention to training and staffing is essential, along with maintenance of skills and continuous quality assessment and improvement.

The important steps in the effective reprocessing of GI endoscopes include:

1. Manual cleaning
2. High-level disinfection
3. Rinsing
4. Drying/appropriate storage.

Effective reprocessing of GI endoscopes is achievable through strict adherence to published guidelines. These standards are best summarized in the Multi-Society Reprocessing Guidelines published in 2003.[2,23] An update to these guidelines is expected in 2010. Transmission of infection through inadequately reprocessed endoscopes is caused by:

- Inadequate manual cleaning
- Inadequate disinfectant or germicidal concentration
- Use of a final rinse with tap water or without adequate drying
- Poor compliance with reprocessing recommendations.

Most cases of transmission of infection by GI endoscopy have resulted from a failure or breakdown in the manual cleaning of the endoscope.[24] Endoscopes that use disposable sheaths and/or valves may provide an alternative to conventional liquid chemical disinfection.

Manual Cleaning

The initial step in endoscopic disinfection, mechanical cleaning, is the most critical.[25–27] Mechanical cleaning leads to removal of a significant amount of organisms, feces, and foreign material from the endoscope. It is important to recall that used endoscopes may have cracks and irregularities, where debris may tend to accumulate during a procedure. Manual cleaning is completed immediately after withdrawal of the endoscope from the patient and is usually done with water, brushing, and/or enzymatic detergents. Washing of the exterior of the endoscope and washing or brushing the interior channels and valves prevents buildup of organic debris and decreases the bioburden, or degree of microbial contamination, in GI endoscopes by 4 logs, or 99.99%.[28–31]

The importance of the manual cleaning step is widely acknowledged in all published guidelines and cannot be overemphasized. Without adequate manual cleaning, retained biofilm on the surface or in the channel of the endoscope can prevent further adequate disinfection, regardless of the method used.[29] Biofilm has been shown to occur in endoscopes as a result of inadequate cleaning, disinfection, rinsing, drying, and storage.[32] All subsequent steps in the reprocessing of an endoscope first require meticulous cleaning of the internal and external surfaces. A survey by Cheung and colleagues[33] in 1999 reported that 9.3% of reporting centers failed to brush the accessory or suction channel, brush the valves, or suction cleaning solution through the endoscope. These results were largely unchanged from a similar survey done in 1995.[34]

High-Level Disinfection

High-level disinfection is the current standard for the reprocessing of endoscopes. It is defined as the destruction of all microorganisms (vegetative bacteria, viruses, fungi, mycobacteria, and some, but not all, bacterial spores). An alternative definition of high-level disinfection is a reduction in the bacterial concentration of 10^6, or 6 logs. This reduction may be achieved through the use of automated endoscope reprocessors (AERs) or by manual reprocessing. Sterilization of an endoscope, while possible using ethylene oxide, is not recommended at present for general endoscopic procedures because there are no data supporting decreased infections, improved safety, or better outcomes as compared with high-level disinfection. High-level disinfection requires complete immersion of the endoscope in the disinfecting solution under specified conditions. The use of endoscopes that cannot be fully immersed is unacceptable.

LCGs for high-level disinfection have been approved for use by the US Food and Drug Administration agency (FDA) (**Table 2**).[35] Such LCGs may be used in both manual and automated reprocessing techniques. Glutaraldehyde ($\geq 2.4\%$ concentration) remains the most commonly used LCG. Other commonly used LCGs include hydrogen peroxide 7.5%, peracetic acid 0.2%, ortho-phthalaldehyde 0.55%, and peracetic acid 0.08% with hydrogen peroxide 1.0%.[35,36] Disinfecting solutions used earlier such as hypochlorite solutions, alcohol, quaternary ammonium compounds, phenolics, and iodophors may not be efficacious, and their use is discouraged.

Many standards recommend that after an endoscope has been mechanically cleaned, high-level disinfection may be achieved by immersion in 2.4% glutaraldehyde for at least 20 minutes at 20°C.[37] This procedure is in conflict with the product labeling. In 1993, the FDA assumed jurisdiction over the regulation of clinical germicides and at that time required manufacturers of 2.4% glutaraldehyde (as part of the 510[k]-clearance process for medical devices) to label their product recommending 45 minutes of exposure to glutaraldehyde at 25°C. This recommendation was based on the length of time and temperature needed for glutaraldehyde to kill 100% of *Mycobacterium tuberculosis* without any manual precleaning.[38] Recognizing the crucial role of mechanical cleaning, subsequent guidelines have suggested that once recommended precleaning has been done, 20 minutes of glutaraldehyde immersion at room temperature is sufficient to achieve high-level disinfection. Current multisociety guidelines reflect this thinking.[2] Glutaraldehyde is currently used in 67% of units at 2.4% concentration; 3.4% glutaraldehyde is used in another 13% of units. In addition, 84% of reporting centers use a "20-minute soak time" technique, and only 24% of centers heat their glutaraldehyde solution.[39]

Potency testing is crucial to the successful use of LCGs and is further discussed later.

Automated Endoscope Reprocessors

Many endoscopy units now use AERs as part of their disinfection procedure. However, the use of an AER does not eliminate the need for manual cleaning.[39,40] Despite the popularity of automated reprocessors, studies have not shown a clear advantage for automated reprocessors over manual high-level disinfection.[41] Automated reprocessors offer potential advantages such as decreased exposure of personnel to LCGs, standardization of the disinfection process, and a reduction in

Table 2
Liquid chemical sterilants used in high-level disinfection in reprocessing of GI endoscopes

Liquid Chemical Sterilant	Advantages	Disadvantages
Glutaraldehyde	Relatively inexpensive Compatible with endoscope materials Long history of use	Vapors cause respiratory irritation Requires ventilation Can fix debris if inadequate cleaning
Hydrogen peroxide	Effective at room temperature No activation needed No odor	May be incompatible with some materials May cause eye damage if contacted Longer contact time
Peracetic acid	Single use Labeled for sterilization Rapidly sporicidal	Relatively expensive May be incompatible with some materials No demonstrated advantage to high-level disinfection
Peracetic acid/ Hydrogen peroxide	No activation required No odor	May be incompatible with some materials Limited clinical experience
Ortho- phthalaldehyde	Rapidly tuberculocidal No odor No activation Effective at room temperature	May require ventilation because of odors May cause staining of clothes Limited clinical experience

Data from Rutula WA, Weber DJ. Disinfection of endoscopes: review of new chemical sterilants used for high-level disinfection. Infect Control Hosp Epidemiol 1999;20:69–76.

manual labor for the staff. Disadvantages include higher cost, inability to disinfect narrow channels (elevator in duodenoscopes), and possibly increased reprocessing time.[42] There has been a significant increase in the use of automated reprocessors over time (69.9% vs 41.5%).[39] Of note, one-third of respondents reported problems with automated reprocessors, including breakdowns, leaks, and damage to endoscopes.[39]

Rinsing

Rinsing the endoscope thoroughly after reprocessing with an LCG is critical in preventing residual germicide from contacting the GI mucosa of subsequent patients. The channels and the endoscope's external surface should be rinsed with copious amounts of water.[2] Glutaraldehyde colitis is a well-recognized phenomenon, and may occur rapidly after exposure of a patient to glutaraldehyde.[43] Hydrogen peroxide exposure to the colonic mucosa leads to a characteristic "snow-white" sign.[44] Recommendations for rinsing suggest that it is done with filtered (through 0.2-μm pores) or sterile water to decrease the risk of microorganisms being reintroduced into the endoscope after high-level disinfection has been completed. Tap water may contain *Pseudomonas*, mycobacteria, or other microorganisms.[45]

Drying/Storage

The final step in the reprocessing procedure is drying, using 70% to 90% ethyl or isopropyl alcohol and forced air drying. This step eliminates residual water that may be trapped in the channels of the endoscope, where such standing water may provide a suitable environment for the multiplication of microorganisms. Although the need for thorough drying after reprocessing is not stressed in all guidelines, many consider this step as important to the prevention of nosocomial infection as cleaning and high-level disinfection.[46]

Endoscopes should be stored without coiling (again to prevent possible pooling of residual water) in a well-ventilated closet.[2]

Some guidelines, including those from the European Society of Gastroenterology and the AORN, suggest the need for reprocessing the endoscopes before the first case of the day. Several studies have concluded that when reprocessed according to established guidelines and stored properly, flexible endoscopes remain free from pathogens overnight and for at least 7 days; according to ASGE and SGNA statements, the practice of additional reprocessing before the first case of the day for endoscopes that have been reprocessed within 10 to 14 days is unnecessary. The interval remains poorly defined and warrants further study.[47–49]

RELATED ISSUES IN REPROCESSING

Several other issues in reprocessing are also relevant to endoscopic practice. Water bottles have been implicated as the source of some pathogen outbreaks (especially *Pseudomonas*) and should be cleaned by high-level disinfection or sterilized at least daily, and sterile water should be used to fill the water bottle.[50]

High-level disinfectants/sterilants must be tested for potency regularly because they become diluted with repeated use. Regular monitoring of the high-level disinfectant/sterilant is mandatory to ensure that the concentration of the active ingredient remains above the minimum effective concentration for germicidal activity. Chemical indicators such as test strips are typically used for this purpose. These indicators must be used in accordance with manufacturer's recommendations to be certain that the chosen high-level disinfectant/sterilant will be effective. Moreover, high-level disinfectants/sterilants have a shelf or reuse life and must be discarded at the end of this reuse life, regardless of the minimal effective concentration. If additional high-level disinfectant/sterilant is added to an AER or manual disinfection basin, the reuse life should be determined by the first use of the original solution (ie, "topping off" does not extend the reuse life of the high-level disinfectant/sterilant).[3,25]

Although everyone involved in endoscopy should be familiar with the essentials of reprocessing, the task of endoscope reprocessing should be the domain of trained staff who regularly perform this function. These personnel should receive device-specific reprocessing instructions to ensure proper cleaning and high-level disinfection, along with regular competency testing to ensure maintenance of skills. Reprocessing should not be assigned to temporary personnel unfamiliar with the equipment and procedures until competence has been established and documented. In addition to having adequately trained staff, attention must be paid to having adequate staffing levels at all times and the scheduling of appropriately trained personnel. Standardization of procedures is critical, and variations from established reprocessing protocols are not acceptable.[2]

REQUIREMENTS FOR THE AMBULATORY SURGERY CENTER, OFFICE ENDOSCOPY, AND HOSPITAL ENDOSCOPY UNIT: DOCUMENTATION AND QUALITY ASSURANCE

Facilities where colonoscopy is performed must meet standards of accrediting organizations; in general, infection-control policies and procedures must be specified, regularly reviewed, and updated as necessary. Written reprocessing protocols should be in place in all facilities where colonoscopy is performed. Regular competency testing of reprocessing personnel should occur.

In addition, a method of tracking each procedure and the endoscope that was used should be in place to assist in an outbreak investigation if one were to occur. Log books or computerized records tracking patients, endoscopes, and AERs used are recommended. Quality assurance programs to verify the effectiveness of all infection-control procedures in endoscopy are important and should be in place in all facilities.[25,27]

SUMMARY

To reduce the risk of infection in colonoscopy, all patients must be considered to be a potential source of infection, and all endoscopes must be reprocessed in a standardized fashion. It is critical to understand that all cases of pathogen transmission related to endoscopy since the advent of guidelines has been the result of a breach in following the accepted protocol. Meticulous attention in following protocols is crucial. Variations to reprocessing protocols are not acceptable; the same procedures are universally applicable in all settings and are critical to assuring a safe procedure.

REFERENCES

1. Everhart JE. The burden of digestive disease in the United States. Bethesda (MA): US Department of Health and Human Services. NIH Publication No 09-6443; 2008.
2. American Society for Gastrointestinal Endoscopy. Multi-society guideline for reprocessing flexible gastrointestinal endoscopes. Gastrointest Endosc 2003;58:1.
3. ASGE Standards of Practice Committee, Banerjee S, Shen B, et al. Infection control during GI endoscopy. Gastrointest Endosc 2008;67:781–90.
4. CDC Guidelines. Available at: http://www.cdc.gov/ncidod/dhqp/gl_isolation.html. Accessed May 5, 2010.
5. OSHA Guidelines. Available at: http://www.osha.gov/SLTC/etools/hospital/hazards/bbp/bbp.html#Uprecautions. Accessed December 14, 2009.
6. Centers for Disease Control and Prevention (CDC). Acute hepatitis C virus infections attributed to unsafe injection practices at an endoscopy clinic—Nevada, 2007. MMWR 2008;57(19):513–7.
7. Nelson DB. Recent advances in epidemiology and prevention of gastrointestinal endoscopy related infections. Curr Opin Infect Dis 2005;18(4):326–30.
8. Rutala WA, Weber DJ. Disinfection and sterilization in health care facilities: what clinicians need to know. Clin Infect Dis 2004;39(5):702–9.
9. DiMarino AJ. Non compliance with FDA and society guidelines for endoscopic reprocessing: Implications for patient care. Gastrointest Endosc Clin N Am 2000; 10:283–94.
10. Nelson DB. Infectious disease complications of GI endoscopy: part II, exogenous infections. Gastrointest Endosc 2003;57(6):695–711.
11. Kimmey MB, Burnett DA, Carr-Locke DL, et al. Transmission of infection by gastrointestinal endoscopy. Gastrointest Endosc 1993;36:885–8.
12. Spach DH, Silverstein FE, Stamm WE. Transmission of infection by gastrointestinal endoscopy and bronchoscopy. Ann Intern Med 1993;118:117–28.
13. Cleaning and disinfection of equipment for gastrointestinal endoscopy. Report of a Working Party of the British Society of Gastroenterology Endoscopy Committee. Gut 1998;42(4):585–93.

14. American Society for Gastrointestinal Endoscopy. Infection control during gastro-intestinal endoscopy: guidelines for clinical application. Gastrointest Endosc 1988;34:37S–40S.
15. Nelson DB, Muscarella LF. Current issues in endoscope reprocessing and infection control during gastrointestinal endoscopy. World J Gastroenterol 2006;12: 3953–64.
16. Chiarello LA. Preventing patient to patient transmission of blood-borne pathogens in health care settings. Semin Infect Contr 2001;1:43–7.
17. Schembre DB. Infectious complications associated with gastrointestinal endoscopy. Gastrointest Endosc Clin N Am 2000;10:215–32.
18. Zubarik R, Fleischer DE, Mastropietro C. Prospective analysis of complications 30 days after outpatient colonoscopy. Gastrointest Endosc 1999;50:322–8.
19. SGNA Guidelines. Standards of infection control in reprocessing of flexible gastrointestinal endoscopes. 2008. Available at: http://www.sgna.org/Resources/3_stdofinfectionFINAL1208_2.pdf. Accessed May 5, 2010.
20. American Society for Testing and Materials. Standard practice for cleaning and disinfection of flexible fiberoptic and video endoscopes used in the examination of the hollow viscera. West Conshohocken (PA): American Society for Testing and Materials; 2000. F1518-00.
21. Association of Perioperative Registered Nurses. Recommended practices for use and care of endoscopes: 2002 standards, recommended practices, and guidelines. Denver (CO): Association of Perioperative Registered Nurses; 2002. p. 229–32.
22. Beilenhoff U, Neumann CS, Rey JF, et al. European Society of Gastrointestinal Endoscopy; European Society of Gastroenterology and Endoscopy Nurses and Associates. ESGE-ESGENA guideline: cleaning and disinfection in gastrointestinal endoscopy. Endoscopy 2008;40:939–57.
23. Rutula WA, Weber DJ. Reprocessing endoscopes: United States perspective. J Hosp Infect 2004;56(Suppl 2):S27–39.
24. Seoane-Vazquez E, Rodriguez-Monnguio R, Visaria J. Endoscopy-related infections and toxic reactions: an international comparison. Endoscopy 2007;39: 742–78.
25. Rutala WA, Weber DJ, The Healthcare Infection Control Practices Advisory Committee (HICPAC). Guideline for disinfection and sterilization in healthcare facilities. 2008. Available at: www.cdc.gov/ncidod/dhqp/pdf/guidelines/Disinfection_Nov_2008.pdf. Accessed November 5, 2009.
26. Banerjee S, Shen B, Nelson DB, et al. Infection control during GI endoscopy. Gastrointest Endosc 2008;67(6):781–90.
27. Society of Gastroenterology Nurses and Associates. Standards of infection control in reprocessing of flexible gastrointestinal endoscopes. Gastroenterol Nurs 2006;29(2):142–8.
28. Chu NS, Favero M. The microbial flora of the gastrointestinal tract and the cleaning of flexible endoscopes. Gastrointest Endosc Clin N Am 2000;20:233–44.
29. Chaufour X, Deva AK, Vickery K, et al. Evaluation of disinfection and sterilization of reusable angioscopes with the duck hepatitis B model. J Vasc Surg 1999;30: 277–82.
30. Vesley D, Melson J, Stanley P. Microbial bioburden in endoscope reprocessing and an in-use evaluation of the high-level disinfection capabilities of Cidex PA. Gastroenterol Nurs 1999;22:63–8.
31. Alfa MJ, Degagne P, Olson N. Worst-case soiling levels for patient-used flexible endoscopes before and after cleaning. Am J Infect Control 1999;27:392–401.

32. Miner N, Harris V, Ebron T, et al. Sporicidal activity of disinfectants as one possible cause for bacteria in patient ready endoscopes. Gastroenterol Nurs 2007;30:285–90.
33. Cheung RJ, Ortiz D, Di Marino AJ. GI endoscopic reprocessing practices in the United States. Gastrointest Endosc 1999;50:362–8.
34. DiMarino AJ. The prevention of infection following gastrointestinal endoscopy: the importance of prophylaxis and reprocessing. In: DiMarino AJ, Benjamin SB, editors. Gastrointestinal disease: an endoscopic approach, vol. 1. 1st edition. (MA): Blackwell Science; 1997. p. 93–104.
35. Rutala WA, Weber DJ. Disinfection of endoscopes: review of new chemical sterilants used for high-level disinfection. Infect Control Hosp Epidemiol 1999;20: 69–76.
36. SGNA standards. Guideline for the use of high-level disinfectants and sterilants for reprocessing of flexible gastrointestinal endoscopes. Gastroenterol Nurs 2000;23:180–7.
37. Rutula WA, Weber DJ. FDA labeling requirements for disinfection of endoscopes: a counterpoint. Infect Control Hosp Epidemiol 1995;16:231–5.
38. Alvarado C. Reconciliation of FDA and societal guidelines for endoscope reprocessing. Gastrointest Endosc Clin N Am 2000;20:275–82.
39. American Society for Gastrointestinal Endoscopy. Technology status evaluation report: automatic endoscope reprocessors. Gastrointest Endosc 1999;50:925–7.
40. Mucarella LF. Automatic flexible endoscope reprocessors. Gastrointest Endosc Clin N Am 2000;10:45–57.
41. Fraser VJ, Zuckerman G, Clouse RE, et al. A prospective, randomized trial comparing manual and automated endoscope disinfection methods. Infect Control Hosp Epidemiol 1993;14:383–9.
42. Muscarella LF. Advantages and limitations of automatic flexible endoscope reprocessors. Am J Infect Control 1996;24:304–9.
43. Farina A, Fievet MH, Plassart F, et al. Residual glutaraldehyde levels in fiberoptic endoscopes: measurement and implications for patient toxicity. J Hosp Infect 1999;42:293–7.
44. Bilotta JJ, Waye JD. Hydrogen peroxide enteritis: the "snow white" sign. Gastrointest Endosc 1989;35:428–30.
45. Muscarella LF. Application of environmental sampling to flexible endoscope reprocessing: the importance of monitoring the rinse water. Infect Control Hosp Epidemiol 2002;23:285–9.
46. Muscarella LF. Inconsistencies in endoscope-reprocessing and infection control guidelines: the importance of endoscope drying. Am J Gastroenterol 2006;101: 2147–54.
47. Osborne S, Reynolds S, George N, et al. Challenging endoscopy reprocessing guidelines: a prospective study investigating the safe shelf life of flexible endoscopes in a tertiary gastroenterology unit. Endoscopy 2007;39:825–30.
48. Rejchrt S, Cermak P, Pavlatova L, et al. Bacteriologic testing of endoscopes after high-level disinfection. Gastrointest Endosc 2004;60:76–8.
49. Vergis AS, Thomson D, Pieroni P, et al. Reprocessing flexible gastrointestinal endoscopes after a period of disuse: is it necessary? Endoscopy 2007;39:737–9.
50. SGNA Practice Committee. Reprocessing of water bottles used during endoscopy. J SGNA 2006;29(5):396–7.

Sedation Issues in Quality Colonoscopy

Lawrence B. Cohen, MD*

KEYWORDS

- Colonoscopy • Sedation • Endoscopic sedation
- Sedation for colonoscopy

Endoscopic sedation for colonoscopy continues to be a controversial issue because of unresolved questions concerning the benefits, risks, and cost of services. Disagreement also exists regarding the most appropriate drug(s), delegation of responsibility for drug administration, patient monitoring, and training qualifications. Sedation is intended to reduce anxiety and discomfort, improve patient tolerability and satisfaction, minimize risk of physical injury, and provide an optimal environment for a thorough examination of the colon. However, it also adds risk, increases cost, slows patient recovery and discharge, increases the amount of time patients lose from work or other activities, and necessitates the presence of an escort upon discharge. This article examines recent trends in endoscopic sedation; evaluates the impact of sedation on the quality, safety, and tolerability of colonoscopy; and reviews the economic implications of current sedation practices.

SEDATION FOR COLONOSCOPY: AN INTERNATIONAL PERSPECTIVE

The variation in sedation practices worldwide reflects the diversity of social, cultural, medicolegal, economic, and market factors that influence patient tolerance for colonoscopy as well as the willingness and ability of endoscopists to expend the time, effort, and resources required for the safe and effective use of sedation. In the United States, the use of endoscopic sedation has been standard practice during endoscopy since the introduction of fiber-optic gastroscopy in the early 1950s. Today, more than 98% of all colonoscopies in the United States are performed with either moderate sedation or monitored anesthesia care (MAC).[1]

In Europe, sedation practices have evolved during the past decade. For example, a study in 1999 indicated that most colonoscopies in Germany were performed without intravenous sedation.[2] Less than 10 years later, a publication by the German Society for Digestive and Metabolic Diseases indicated that the use of intravenous sedation during colonoscopy in that country was nearly 88%.[3] A similar trend has been observed in Switzerland, where the use of sedation during colonoscopy increased from 60% to

Disclosures: None relevant to the content of this article.
Mount Sinai School of Medicine, New York, NY 10029, USA
* New York Gastroenterology Associates, 311 East 79th Street, Suite 2A, New York, NY 10075.
E-mail address: lawrence.cohen@nyga.md

Gastrointest Endoscopy Clin N Am 20 (2010) 615–627
doi:10.1016/j.giec.2010.07.003
1052-5157/10/$ – see front matter © 2010 Elsevier Inc. All rights reserved.

78% between 1990 and 2003.[4] During this time, the average number of colonoscopies performed annually by a Swiss endoscopist increased nearly 60%. Most of these colonoscopies were performed using a benzodiazepine and an opioid, although 34% of endoscopists indicated that they routinely administered propofol. The use of propofol by endoscopists in Germany is also growing, according to anecdotal reports.

Sedation practices vary considerably throughout Europe, however. In 2007, a survey of 278 centers throughout Italy reported that sedation was used during 55% of colonoscopies. The methods of sedation included benzodiazepine alone (28%), benzodiazepine and opioid (15%), propofol (3%), and other method of sedation (8%).[5] In 2008, a survey of 197 endoscopy centers in Spain indicated that most used sedation for at least 50% of their colonoscopies.[6] The agents used included benzodiazepine alone (13%), benzodiazepine and opioid (39%), opioid alone (15%), propofol (21%), and unspecified (12%). A nationwide survey of Greek endoscopists in 2007 found that 78% of respondents used intravenous sedation routinely during colonoscopy.[7] Unsedated colonoscopy is increasingly uncommon in Europe, according to a recent survey that found it to be the dominant method of sedation in only 5 European countries: Norway, Poland, Russia, Serbia, and Montenegro.[8]

The data available regarding sedation practices in Asia and Africa are sparse. Anecdotal information based on surveys of small numbers of individuals practicing within these 2 continents indicates that the use of sedation varies considerably from country to country. For example, the use of sedation during colonoscopy in Asia ranged between 0% and 100% of cases, with the highest use rates in Australia and Hong Kong (100%), and the lowest rates in China and Taiwan (0%–15%).[9] A similar situation exists in Africa, where sedation use is closely linked to the economic environment of the individual practice and the country. Among 13 African endoscopy units that were surveyed, 100% responded that sedation was administered during most colonoscopies. In most instances, midazolam was used alone, although almost half of those surveyed indicated that propofol was used in some cases.[9] Benson and colleagues[8] reported similar findings regarding sedation practices in Africa and Asia, based on a survey of 165 endoscopists practicing worldwide.

In summary, the administration of sedation during colonoscopy has evolved during the past decade. Today, relatively few countries exist where most examinations are performed without sedation. In spite of cultural, social, and medicolegal differences that exist from one region to another, market demand and economic considerations are the dominant forces influencing the practice of sedation during colonoscopy.

THE ECONOMIC IMPLICATIONS OF SEDATION

Historically, sedation has been the responsibility of the endoscopist, assisted by a nurse or endoscopy technician. The administration of moderate sedation involves a variety of tasks including the pre-procedure evaluation, establishment of intravenous access and delivery of fluids, administration of intravenous medications, patient monitoring both during and after the procedure, recovery assessment, and patient discharge. Additional sedation-related functions include documentation, maintenance of emergency equipment, and medication inventory. It has been estimated that this work, combined with the practice expense of sedation, account for up to 40% of the total overhead cost of an endoscopic examination.[10] With estimates of the direct overhead cost of colonoscopy ranging from $200 to $400, the approximate cost of providing moderate sedation works out to $80 to $160 per procedure.[11,12]

Reimbursement for the cost of sedation is bundled into the professional fee for endoscopy, according to Appendix G of the American Medical Association's Current

Procedural Terminology (CPT).[13] Consequently, when an endoscopist performs sedation during an endoscopic procedure, a separate charge for this service is not permitted under Centers for Medicare and Medicaid Services (CMS) policy. Many commercial payers, following the lead of CMS, have also adopted this policy.

The value that CMS has placed on sedation services cannot be accurately determined, as the endoscopic CPT codes include no relative value units for the physician work that is directly attributed to sedation administration. New CPT codes for moderate sedation (99143-99145) were established in 2006 for instances in which the provider of sedation also performed the diagnostic or therapeutic procedure. However, CMS policy precludes the use of these codes for procedures listed in Appendix G, which encompasses all of the endoscopic procedures. Moreover, CMS deems these codes to be carrier priced, and has not established relative value units for these services.

The exclusion of sedation as a unique service for procedures listed within Appendix G does not apply to anesthesia services. Complex procedures and procedures in high-risk patients are considered circumstances in which the presence of an anesthesia specialist is considered necessary and appropriate. A statement issued jointly by the American Gastroenterological Association (AGA), the American College of Gastroenterology (ACG), and the American Society for Gastrointestinal Endoscopy (ASGE) supports this conclusion, indicating that the routine use of an anesthesiologist for average-risk patients undergoing standard upper and lower endoscopic procedures is not warranted (**Box 1**). That notwithstanding, the use of anesthesia services in the United States has grown considerably during the past decade. Estimates suggest that an anesthesia provider is involved in 30% or more of all endoscopic procedures, and this number is projected to grow by 20% or so annually during the next several years.[14] Similar changes have been observed in some provinces of Canada. For example, the proportion of colonoscopies in Ontario involving an anesthesiologist increased from 8% to 19% between 1993 and 2005.[15] The economic impact of this trend is considerable. If sedation were to be provided by an anesthesiologist for all colonoscopies performed in the United States, which now exceed 15 million annually, the cost for this service would exceed $7.2 billion a year! This figure is based on an average reimbursement rate of $480 per case for anesthesia services. The potential economic and clinical consequences of this additional expense on the practice of gastroenterology, and colonoscopy in particular, have been reviewed in detail in several recent articles.[16,17]

Traditionally, anesthesiologists performing ambulatory anesthesia for endoscopy have billed independently for their services. In some areas of the country, it is routine for the anesthesiologist to be nonparticipating in health insurance plans even though the endoscopist and the facility may be in-network. Under such an arrangement, it would not be unusual for the endoscopist to be paid $500 to $600 for performing a colonoscopy, whereas the anesthesiologist is reimbursed as much as $1000 or more. A recent review of this subject indicated that the commercial anesthesia fee for lower endoscopy (CPT code 00810) is 60% higher than the endoscopist's fee (CPT code 45378), based on the relative value units for each code.[18]

This disparity in compensation has prompted some endoscopists and facility owners to develop alternative business models to capture some of the revenue generated by anesthesia services. One approach that has been used is renting or leasing space, equipment, and/or personnel to the anesthesia group, or by charging for billing and collection services. Provided that the charges are set at fair market value, such an arrangement would qualify for safe harbor protection and would not be construed as a kickback. If the group is charged above-market rates, however, it is very possible

---

Box 1

American Gastroenterological Association, American College of Gastroenterology, and American Society for Gastrointestinal Endoscopy recommendations on the administration of sedation for the performance of endoscopic procedures

- In general, diagnostic and uncomplicated therapeutic endoscopy and colonoscopy are successfully performed with moderate (conscious) sedation.
- Compared with standard doses of benzodiazepines and narcotics, propofol provides faster onset and deeper sedation.
- More rapid cognitive and functional recovery can be expected with the use of propofol as a single agent.
- Clinically important benefits over standard sedation have not been consistently demonstrated in average-risk patients undergoing routine upper and lower endoscopy. Further randomized clinical trials are needed in this setting.
- Propofol may have clinically significant advantages when used for prolonged and therapeutic procedures, including, but not limited to, endoscopic retrograde cholangiopancreatography and endoscopic ultrasound.
- There are data to support the use of propofol by adequately trained nonanesthesiologists. Large case series indicate that with adequate training, physician-supervised nurse administration of propofol can be done safely and effectively. The regulations governing the administration of propofol by nursing personnel vary from state to state.
- Patients receiving propofol should receive care consistent with deep sedation. Personnel should be capable of rescuing the patients from general anesthesia and/or severe respiratory depression.
- A designated individual, other than the endoscopist, should be present to monitor the patient throughout the procedure and should be able to recognize and assist in the management of complications.
- The routine assistance of an anesthesiologist/anesthetist for average-risk patients undergoing standard upper and lower endoscopic procedures is not warranted.
- Physician-nurse teams administering propofol should possess the training and skills necessary to rescue patients from severe respiratory depression.
- Complex procedures and procedures in high-risk patients may justify the use of an anesthesiologist/anesthetist to provide conscious and/or deep sedation. In such cases, this provider may bill separately for professional services.
- The use of agents to achieve sedation for endoscopy must conform to the policies of the individual institution.
- Reimbursement for conscious sedation is included within the codes covering endoscopic sedation.
- Billing separately for conscious sedation has been targeted by the Office of Inspector General as a possible fraud and abuse violation, and is not recommended.

Data from Joint Statement of a Working Group from the American College of Gastroenterology, the American Gastroenterological Association and the American Society for Gastrointestinal endoscopy. Recommendations on the administration of sedation for the performance of endoscopic procedures. Available at: http://www.gastro.org/wmspage.cfm?parm1=371 2004. Accessed August 14, 2006.

---

that the excess payment would be characterized as a kickback, which was provided in exchange for the right to provide anesthesia services.

Recently, some ambulatory endoscopy centers have shifted to an "in-house model," which involves contracting with or hiring an anesthesia provider. In this model, the anesthesia provider becomes an employee of the facility or practice and is paid a salary for his or her services. The facility then bills and retains the professional fees for the anesthesia services. Under such an arrangement, some payers may decline to reimburse a facility fee as well as payment for the anesthesia professional services under a single tax identification number.

An alternative to the in-house model is the "company model," whereby either the physician practice or facility forms a new company (an anesthesia services company) for the explicit purpose of employing anesthesia providers, either anesthesiologists or certified registered nurse anesthetists. The anesthesia services company bills for the anesthesia services and pays a salary to the providers, and the profits from this company are shared by the company's owners. Some estimates place the distributed profits at 40% or more of the anesthesia fees. Because the owners of the anesthesia company do not have to be the same individuals who own the practice or facility, this model provides an opportunity to select only those individuals who should be involved in this ancillary business activity, rather than dividing the profits among all owners of the facility or practice. From a regulatory perspective, the status of the company model remains uncertain, as the arrangement could be viewed as a contractual joint arrangement under the federal antikickback statute. The American Society of Anesthesiology (ASA) has requested the Office of Inspector General to issue a Special Advisory Bulletin clarifying the legality of the company model, but the status of this request remains uncertain at the time of writing.

What conclusions can be drawn from the preceding analysis? First, reimbursement for sedation administered by an endoscopist is insufficient to cover the cost of providing this service. Although most endoscopists in the United States continue to administer sedation, this imbalance between cost and reimbursement remains a powerful motivation for an ever-growing number of endoscopists to involve an anesthesia provider. Second, anesthesiologist-assisted endoscopy offers several benefits to the endoscopist, including the remarkable drug propofol, the services of an additional medical provider, and, in some instances, added revenue for the practice or facility. Third, the presence of a second provider for sedation adds considerably to the cost of colonoscopy with little or no improvement in the quality or safety. In a recent editorial in *Anesthesiology*, Orkin and Duncan[19] referred to this practice as an example "in which low-benefit services and procedures result in disproportionate expenditures… [and] … are ideal substrate for health care reform." To address these issues, we must reexamine and modify the current system of coding and reimbursement for procedural sedation. Changes to be considered include (1) a revision of payment levels for procedural sedation to better align compensation with the work and practice expenses associated with this service, (2) a reduction in professional fees for proceduralists who delegate sedation to a second provider, and (3) the development of guidelines that define those procedures and patients in whom the involvement of an anesthesiologist is medically appropriate.

SEDATION AND THE QUALITY OF COLONOSCOPY

Based on clinical experience, most endoscopists believe that sedation improves the quality of colonoscopy. Unfortunately, few studies have systematically examined this issue. A recent review of the literature failed to uncover a single randomized controlled study designed and powered to demonstrate a difference in the quality of sedated versus unsedated colonoscopy.[20] Nonrandomized observational and cohort studies are available, however, that contribute to our understanding of endoscopic sedation and its impact on the quality of colonoscopy.

The role of sedation on the technical performance of colonoscopy was examined by Radaelli and colleagues.[21] A total of 278 practice sites throughout Italy were prospectively evaluated over a 2-week period. Cecal intubation and polyp detection rates were assessed in 12,835 colonoscopies. Sedation was used during colonoscopy in 55.3% of cases, whereas the remaining cases were performed without sedation. The methods of sedation included a benzodiazepine alone (28.8%), a benzodiazepine plus an opioid (15.4%), propofol (3.1%), and other sedation regimens (7.5%). Other variables that were examined included quality of bowel preparation, procedure setting, endoscopist, patient age and gender, procedure indication, and endoscopic complications. The overall rate of cecal intubation was 80.7% of cases, including 76.1% of unsedated and 84.2% of sedated procedures. Compared with procedures performed without sedation, the use of a benzodiazepine increased the likelihood of reaching the cecum by 46%, and the combination of a benzodiazepine and an opioid (odds ratio [OR] 2.1, 95% confidence interval [CI] 1.7–2.5) or propofol (OR 2.4, 95% CI 1.6–3.5) further increased the rate of cecal intubation. Intravenous sedation also increased the likelihood of identifying at least one polyp (OR 1.17, 95% CI 1.0–1.2). The use of a benzodiazepine alone, a benzodiazepine plus an opioid, and propofol were all associated with an increased probability of polyp detection (11%, 12%, and 32%, respectively), compared with those procedures that were performed without sedation.

Conigliaro and Rossi[22] reported the findings of an observational study that compared the quality of examination and cecal intubation rates between sedated and unsedated patients. Colonoscopy was more likely to be complete in sedated than in unsedated patients ($P<.001$). In contrast, Eckardt and colleagues[2] observed similar rates of cecal intubation among sedated and unsedated patients undergoing colonoscopy (92.5% vs 91.9%, respectively), although polypectomy rates were higher in the sedated group (25.0% vs 16.7%, respectively). Most experts agree that cecal intubation time is prolonged by several minutes in an unsedated colonoscopy, especially if the examination must then be interrupted to administer medication.[23,24]

A recent report from Germany used a national endoscopic database to examine the outcomes of 236,000 routine colonoscopies performed during a 1-year period. Intravenous sedation was used in 92.8% of cases and the cumulative rate of complete colonoscopies was 97.4%.[3] A multivariate logistic regression identified predictors of incomplete colonoscopy, which included sedation and/or analgesia (OR 0.507, 95% CI 0.411–0.626). These findings indicate that the use of sedation/analgesia increased the likelihood of a complete colonoscopy nearly twofold.

On the basis of these observational and cohort studies, it is reasonable to conclude that overall rates of cecal intubation and polyp detection are increased in procedures performed with sedation. Several unanswered questions related to this issue remain, however. Is the success of colonoscopy related to the method of sedation? Do the outcomes of colonoscopy differ with deep sedation compared with moderate sedation? Can we identify a subset of patients in whom unsedated colonoscopy would provide comparable quality to a sedated examination? A recent analysis of a national endoscopic database compared the outcomes of 101,367 colonoscopies performed under moderate sedation with 3501 colonoscopies that were performed under deep sedation. More large colon polyps were found with deep sedation than with moderate sedation (7.2% vs 6.0%, $P = .01$).[25] Unfortunately, serious methodological flaws make the results of this study difficult to interpret. Well-designed randomized controlled studies are necessary to address these and other related issues.

In conclusion, there is increasing evidence that the use of sedation or MAC improves the rates of cecal intubation and polyp detection, 2 quality measures for colonoscopy. There is no evidence to favor one method of sedation compared with another, however. It is likely that similar outcomes can be achieved during unsedated colonoscopy, provided the examiner possesses the necessary skills and patience, and the patient is sufficiently motivated to tolerate some discomfort. The benefits of unsedated colonoscopy include an opportunity for the patient to observe and understand the procedure, and the option of resuming pre-procedure activities with little or no time lost as a result of recovery. Notwithstanding these benefits, most patients undergoing colonoscopy prefer to be sedated for their examination.

DOES SEDATION IMPROVE PATIENT SATISFACTION?

There is widespread agreement among providers and experts in health care outcomes that patient satisfaction is an important measure of success in health care delivery. The ASGE/ACG Taskforce on Quality in Endoscopy proposed that patient satisfaction be considered a quality indicator of endoscopy.[26] Factors that have been demonstrated to influence patient satisfaction during colonoscopy include the endoscopist's personal manner, the nurse's personal manner, the patient's perception of technical skills of the provider, the physical environment, and pain or discomfort during the procedure. That adequate control of discomfort during colonoscopy is among the most important determinants of patient satisfaction has been shown in numerous studies.[27–29]

Sedation reduces discomfort, improves patient tolerance and satisfaction with colonoscopy, and increases compliance with recommendations for subsequent examinations. In a systematic review of 11 colonoscopy trials, McQuaid and Laine[20] observed that 89% of patients sedated with midazolam and a narcotic were satisfied with the sedation, and 82% were willing to repeat the procedure with the same sedation. Fewer than 10% of patients reported pain or nausea, although 36% had some memory of the procedure. Although it is widely thought that the combination of a benzodiazepine and an opioid is superior to either agent alone, there are no randomized studies to support this conclusion.

Propofol is being used increasingly for sedation during colonoscopy.[30,31] Numerous studies have assessed patient satisfaction with propofol compared with standard sedation. The interpretation of these studies is complicated, however, because of significant variations in the methods of propofol administration and the use of nonvalidated instruments for assessing patient satisfaction. For example, propofol may be administered either alone or combined with one or more agents; administered by bolus administration, continuous infusion, or patient-controlled sedation; and targeted to either moderate or deep sedation. Patient satisfaction with propofol sedation has been reported as higher in several studies,[32–34] whereas other studies have found no difference.[35] A pooled analysis of 4 studies using propofol either alone or in combination with another agent observed higher patient satisfaction with use of propofol compared with standard sedation (OR for dissatisfaction 0.42, 95% CI 0.29–0.59).

In addition to minimizing anxiety and procedure-related discomfort, rapid recovery and an ability to resume pre-procedure activities are important elements of patient satisfaction. Published studies indicate that both recovery and discharge times are shorter with the use of propofol compared with traditional sedation. Three of 4 studies comparing propofol alone to traditional sedation observed shorter recovery times with propofol, with a mean difference of 14.7 minutes.[33,35–37] Similarly, 6 of 7 studies comparing propofol in combination with another agent to traditional sedation reported shorter recovery times with propofol (mean difference, 17.9 minutes).[32,38–42]

Of paramount importance to many patients is whether a short-acting agent such as propofol will enable them to resume working and/or driving within a short period of time following the examination. There are relatively few data that address this issue. Ulmer and colleagues[35] compared recovery time and cognitive performance as measured by psychometric tests in subjects undergoing colonoscopy with either standard sedation or propofol. Recovery time was faster with propofol than midazolam and fentanyl (16.5 vs 27.5 minutes, $P = .0001$) and postprocedure tests of verbal learning, memory, visual-motor coordination, and response inhibition were better in the group that received propofol. It has been more challenging to demonstrate a meaningful improvement in functional ability. Two studies have assessed driving ability following recovery from propofol. Riphaus and colleagues[43] compared driving skills as assessed using a driving simulator 2 hours after sedation with either propofol or standard sedation (midazolam and pethidine) in patients undergoing routine esophagogastroduodenoscopy (EGD) or colonoscopy. Driving skills after propofol were virtually unchanged from the baseline measurements, whereas a significant decline in performance was observed in the patients who received standard sedation. Horiuchi and colleagues[44] compared driving performance on a simulator in patients sedated with low-dose propofol either alone or combined with midazolam before EGD. Driving ability returned to baseline levels within 1 hour after propofol but remained impaired at 2 hours after propofol and midazolam. It is important to point out that the average dose of propofol in this study was only 30 to 40 mg. These data clearly indicate that recovery of psychomotor function is faster with propofol than standard sedation. Additional studies are required, however, to determine the time required for complete recovery in all individuals receiving this form of sedation. At the present time it is recommended that patients sedated with propofol avoid driving an automobile for at least 4 hours after the procedure.

Unsedated colonoscopy provides several important benefits for the patient. First, patients not receiving sedation are permitted to resume their normal activities soon after completing their examination. For some patients, this alone is a very compelling reason to favor an unsedated examination. Second, unsedated patients can drive themselves home after an examination and do not require an escort. Third, the risk of sedation-related complications is avoided when performing an unsedated examination. And last, the cost of endoscopy may be significantly reduced if sedation is eliminated. In spite of these benefits, only 2% to 7% of patients undergoing colonoscopy in the United States elect not to receive sedation.[45] Nonetheless, unsedated colonoscopy can be an effective alternative for select patients. In a series of 2090 consecutive outpatients presenting for colonoscopy, Petrini and colleagues[23] completed colonoscopy without sedation in 81.1% of 578 carefully selected patients who opted to undergo an unsedated procedure. Consequently, 22% of this cohort completed their colonoscopy without sedation. Men were more likely than woman to accept unsedated colonoscopy (40.2% vs 16.1%, $P<.001$), and individuals with a history of prior abdominal surgery were less likely to complete the examination without receiving sedation. Moderate or severe pain was more likely to be reported by unsedated than sedated (16% and 23% vs 8% and 22%, respectively, $P<.001$) patients. Nonetheless, in spite of experiencing pain, unsedated male patients were more willing to have another examination performed in the same fashion than patients who received sedation ($P<.001$ for men, $P<.2$ for women).

For most patients, the use of sedation during colonoscopy improves tolerability and satisfaction with the examination, and increases their willingness to undergo a subsequent procedure. Furthermore, satisfactory sedation can usually be achieved with either a benzodiazepine/opioid combination or propofol. The literature indicates that recovery is faster and that fewer sedation-related side effects occur with propofol than under standard sedation, however. Although cognitive function, motor coordination, and driving skills as assessed by simulation have been demonstrated to be normal 2 hours following sedation with propofol, the consensus of opinion remains that patients should be instructed to not drive for the remainder of the day after receiving any form of intravenous sedation.

SEDATION AND THE RISK OF COMPLICATIONS DURING COLONOSCOPY

An endoscopic complication may be defined as an undesired outcome that occurs as a result of a procedure and requires some form of change in the management of the patient.[46] Complications may range in severity from trivial to life-threatening. Although a variety of endoscopic adverse events have been attributed anecdotally to patient sedation, only cardiopulmonary complications have been definitely related to sedation practices. Some investigators have also suggested that the rate of bowel perforation might be affected by the method of sedation. This review evaluates and compares relative rates of cardiopulmonary complications associated with different sedation methods, including unsedated colonoscopy, and also reviews the available literature on bowel perforation and different sedation methods.

The reported rate of colon perforation following colonoscopy ranges from 1 in 500 to less than 1 in 10,000.[3,47–50] Identifiable risk factors for perforation include increased age, comorbid illness, trainee involvement, and endoscopic polypectomy. With one notable exception,[21] published studies have not demonstrated that endoscopic sedation is an independent risk factor for bowel perforation, and a recent comprehensive review of the literature on colonoscopy perforation supports this conclusion.[51]

A related issue is whether the use of propofol increases the risk of perforation compared with standard sedation agents. Previously, several investigators raised concerns that propofol, by reducing patient feedback from a painful stimulus such as excessive stretching or distension of the colon, might increase the risk of creating a tear in the bowel wall.[52] More recent studies, however, indicate that the risk of bowel perforation during colonoscopy is similar irrespective of whether the procedure was performed under standard sedation or propofol.[53–55]

Cardiorespiratory events are observed commonly during colonoscopy. Depending on the definition applied, unplanned cardiopulmonary events occur at a rate of 0.06% to 0.90%. Recognized risk factors for cardiorespiratory complications include patient age, patient ASA physical classification, inpatient status, and trainee involvement with a procedure.[56] In an analysis of the Clinical Outcomes Research Initiative data, Sharma and colleagues[56] observed that the rate of cardiopulmonary events was inversely related to the doses of fentanyl and midazolam that were administered. This suggests that patients with greater sensitivity to sedation and analgesic drugs are at higher risk of developing a cardiopulmonary event. Dosing should therefore be done with small boluses of drug titrated to the desired effect, and the doses separated by sufficient time to avoid a "stacking" effect. The analysis also indicated that use of supplemental oxygen was associated with an increased rate of cardiopulmonary events. That supplemental oxygen delays recognition of hypoventilation is well known, and there is mounting evidence that it impairs the timely detection of hypoventilation or apnea and leads to an increase in sedation-related complications.[57,58]

Not all cardiopulmonary events are associated with the use of sedation. For example, Radaelli and colleagues[5] observed in a large, nationwide survey that serious cardiorespiratory complications necessitating the discontinuation of endoscopy occurred with similar rates in unsedated patients as in those who received sedation.

The comparative safety of standard sedation compared with propofol during endoscopic procedures has been examined in multiple studies. A meta-analysis of these two forms of sedation showed that propofol sedation was associated with a lower odds ratio of major cardiopulmonary complications (defined as hypoxemia, hypotension, arrhythmias, and apnea) during colonoscopy than an opioid and benzodiazepine combination.[59] This finding is supported by a systematic literature review[20] and a Cochrane review,[60] which both concluded that there was no difference in the rate of complications between standard sedation and propofol. Unfortunately, prospective studies comparing the safety of endoscopist-directed sedation, using either a benzodiazepine and opioid or propofol, and monitored anesthesia care have yet to be reported.

SUMMARY

Quality colonoscopy can be achieved either with or without the use of sedation. Unsedated colonoscopy requires that the endoscopist possess patience, skill, and dedication because some unsedated examinations will require additional time. Most endoscopists throughout the world now use sedation for most of the colonoscopies that they perform. Sedation is intended to minimize patient discomfort, increase compliance with colorectal cancer screening and surveillance guidelines, and, in most circumstances, improve the quality of examination. Both cecal intubation and polyp detection rates may be improved with sedation. There is no evidence, however, that indicates that one method of sedation yields better outcomes than any other form of conventional sedation. Additional research is needed to assess the comparative effectiveness of endoscopist- and anesthetist-directed sedation for colonoscopy.

REFERENCES

1. Cohen LB, Wecsler JS, Gaetano JN, et al. Endoscopic sedation in the United States: results from a nationwide survey. Am J Gastroenterol 2006;101(5):967–74.
2. Eckardt VF, Kanzler G, Schmitt T, et al. Complications and adverse effects of colonoscopy with selective sedation. Gastrointest Endosc 1999;49(5):560–5.
3. Crispin A, Birkner B, Munte A, et al. Process quality and incidence of acute complications in a series of more than 230,000 outpatient colonoscopies. Endoscopy 2009;41:1018–25.
4. Heuss LT, Froehlich F, Beglinger C. Changing patterns of sedation and monitoring practice during endoscopy: results of a nationwide survey in Switzerland. Endoscopy 2005;37(2):161–6.
5. Radaelli F, Meucci G, Minoli G. Colonoscopy practices in Italy: a prospective survey on behalf of the Italian Association of Hospital Gastroenterologists. Dig Liver Dis 2008;103:1122–30.
6. Baudet JS, Borque P, Borja E, et al. Use of sedation in gastrointestinal endoscopy: a nationwide survey in Spain. Gastroenterol Hepatol 2009;21:882–8.
7. Paspatis GA, Manolaraki MM, Tribonias G, et al. Endoscopic sedation in Greece: results from a nationwide survey for the Hellenic Foundation of Gastroenterology and Nutrition. Dig Liver Dis 2009;41:807–11.
8. Benson AA, Cohen LB, Waye JD, et al. Endoscopic sedation within developing and developed countries. Gut Liver 2008;2:105–12.
9. Ladas SD, Satake Y, Mostafa I, et al. Sedation practices for gastrointestinal endoscopy in Europe, North America, Asia, Africa and Australia. Digestion 2010;82:74–6.

10. Abraham N, Barkun A, Larocque M, et al. Predicting which patients can undergo upper endoscopy comfortably without conscious sedation. Gastrointest Endosc 2002;56(2):180–9.
11. Sharara N, Adams V, Crott R, et al. The costs of colonoscopy in a Canadian hospital using a microcosting approach. Can J Gastroenterol 2008;22:565–70.
12. Henry SG, Ness RM, Stiles RA, et al. A cost analysis of colonoscopy using microcosting and time-and-motion techniques. J Gen Intern Med 2007;22:1415–21.
13. Beebe M, Dalton JA, Esponceda M. CPT 2009 Professional Edition. Chicago: American Medical Association; 2009.
14. Inadomi JM, Gunnarsson CL, Rizzo JA, et al. Projected growth rate of anesthesiologist-delivered sedation in colonoscopy and EGD in the United States: 2009-2011. Gastrointest Endosc 2009;69:AB111.
15. Alharbi O, Rabeneck L, Paszat LF, et al. A population-based analysis of outpatient colonoscopy in adults assisted by an anesthesiologist. Anesthesiology 2009;111:734–40.
16. Aisenberg J, Brill JV, Ladabaum U, et al. Sedation for gastrointestinal endoscopy: new practices, new economics. Am J Gastroenterol 2005;100(5):996–1000.
17. Rex DK. The science and politics of propofol. Am J Gastroenterol 2004;99(11): 2080–3.
18. Hannenberg AA. Payment for procedural sedation. Curr Opin Anaesthesiol 2004; 17:171–6.
19. Orkin FK, Duncan PG. Substrate for healthcare reform: anesthesia's low-lying fruit. Anesthesiology 2009;111:697–8.
20. McQuaid KR, Laine L. A systematic review and meta-analysis of randomized, controlled trials of moderate sedation for routine endoscopic procedures. Gastrointest Endosc 2008;67:910–23.
21. Radaelli F, Meucci G, Sgroi G, et al. Technical performance of colonoscopy: the key role of sedation/analgesia and other quality indicators. Am J Gastroenterol 2008;103:1122–30.
22. Conigliaro R, Rossi A. Implementation of sedation guidelines in clinical practice in Italy: results of a prospective longitudinal multicenter study. Endoscopy 2006;38: 1137–43.
23. Petrini J, Egan JV, Hanh WV. Unsedated colonoscopy: patient characteristics and satisfaction in a community-based endoscopy unit. Gastrointest Endosc 2009;69: 567–72.
24. Rex DK, Imperiale TF, Portish V. Patients willing to try colonoscopy without sedation: associated clinical factors and results of a randomized controlled trial. Gastrointest Endosc 1999;49(5):554–9.
25. Hoda KM, Holub JL, Eisen GM. More large polyps are seen on screening colonoscopy with deep sedation compared with moderate sedation [abstract]. Gastrointest Endosc 2009;69:AB119–20.
26. Faigel D, Pike IM, Baron JH, et al. Quality indicators for gastrointestinal endoscopic procedures: an introduction. Gastrointest Endosc 2006;63:S3–9.
27. Ko HH, Zhang H, Telford JJ, et al. Factors influencing patient satisfaction when undergoing endoscopic procedures. Gastrointest Endosc 2009;69:883–91.
28. Yacavone RF, Locke GR III, Gostout CJ, et al. Factors influencing patient satisfaction with GI endoscopy. Gastrointest Endosc 2001;53(7):703–10.
29. Subramanian S, Liangpunsakul S, Rex DK. Preprocedure patient values regarding sedation for colonoscopy. J Clin Gastroenterol 2005;39:516–9.
30. Rex DK, Deenadayalu VP, Eid E, et al. Endoscopist-directed administration of propofol: a worldwide safety experience. Gastroenterology 2009;137:1229–37.

31. Vargo JJ, Cohen LB, Rex DK, et al. Position statement: nonanesthesiologist administration of propofol for GI endoscopy. Am J Gastroenterol 2009;104: 2886–92.
32. Reimann FM, Samson U, Derad I, et al. Synergistic sedation with low-dose midazolam and propofol for colonoscopies. Endoscopy 2000;32(3):239–44.
33. Sipe BW, Rex DK, Latinovich D, et al. Propofol versus midazolam/meperidine for outpatient colonoscopy: administration by nurses supervised by endoscopists. Gastrointest Endosc 2002;55(7):815–25.
34. Paspatis GA, Manolaraki M, Xirouchakis G, et al. Synergistic sedation with midazolam and propofol versus midazolam and pethidine in colonoscopies: a prospective, randomized study. Am J Gastroenterol 2002;97(8):1963–7.
35. Ulmer BJ, Hansen JJ, Overley CA, et al. Propofol versus midazolam/fentanyl for outpatient colonoscopy: administration by nurses supervised by endoscopists. Clin Gastroenterol Hepatol 2003;1(6):425–32.
36. Munoz-Navas M, Garcia-Pedrajas F, Panadero A, et al. Midazolam-flumazenil versus propofol for ambulatory colonoscopy. Preliminary results of a randomized single blinded study. Gastrointest Endosc 1994;40:P29.
37. Moerman AT, Foubert LA, Herregods LL, et al. Propofol versus remifentanil for monitored anesthesia care during colonoscopy. Eur J Anaesthesiol 2003;20:461–6.
38. Bright E, Roseveare C, Dalgleish D, et al. Patient-controlled sedation for colonoscopy: a randomized trial comparing patient-controlled administration of propofol and alfentanil with physician-administered midazolam and pethidine. Endoscopy 2003;35(8):683–7.
39. Roseveare C, Seavell C, Patel P, et al. Patient-controlled sedation and analgesia, using propofol and alfentanil, during colonoscopy: a prospective randomized controlled trial. Endoscopy 1998;30(9):768–73.
40. Mandel JE, Tanner JW, Lichtenstein G, et al. A randomized, controlled, double-blind trial of patient-controlled sedation with propofol/remifentanil versus midazolam/fentanyl for colonoscopy. Anesth Analg 2008;106:434–9.
41. Kotash MA, Johnston R, Baily RJ, et al. Sedation for colonoscopy: a double-blind comparison of diazepam/meperidine, midazolam/fentanyl and propofol/fentanyl combinations. Can J Gastroenterol 1994;8:27–31.
42. Liu GM, Ching JY, Chan SK, et al. A randomized trial comparing patient-controlled sedation using propofol/alfentanil to diazemul/pethidine in patients undergoing outpatient colonoscopy [abstract]. Gastrointest Endosc 2000;51:AB62.
43. Riphaus A, Gstettenbauer T, Frenz MB, et al. Quality of psychomotor recovery after propofol sedation for routine endoscopy: a randomized and controlled study. Endoscopy 2006;38(7):677–83.
44. Horiuchi A, Nakayama Y, Katsuyama Y, et al. Safety and driving ability following low-dose propofol sedation. Digestion 2008;78:190–4.
45. Rex DK, Khalfan HK. Sedation and the technical performance of colonoscopy. Gastrointest Endosc Clin N Am 2005;15(4):661–72.
46. Mergener K. Defining and measuring endoscopic complications: more questions than answers. In: Ginsberg GG, editor. Minimizing endoscopic complications. Philadelphia: WB Saunders Company; 2007. p. 1–9.
47. Rabeneck L, Paszat LF, Hilsden RJ, et al. Bleeding and perforation after outpatient colonoscopy and their risk factors in usual clinical practice. Gastroenterology 2008;135:1899–906.
48. Gatto NM, Frucht H, Sundararajan V, et al. Risk of perforation after colonoscopy and sigmoidoscopy: a population-based study. J Natl Cancer Inst 2003;95(3): 230–6.

49. Regula J, Rupinski M, Kraszewska E, et al. Colonoscopy in colorectal cancer screening for detection of advanced neoplasia. N Engl J Med 2006;355:1863–72.
50. Ko CW, Riffle S, Michaels L, et al. Serious complications within 30 days of screening and surveillance colonoscopy are uncommon. Clin Gastroenterol Hepatol 2010;8:166–73.
51. Panteris V, Haringsma J, Kuipers EJ. Colonoscopy perforation rate, mechanisms and outcome: from diagnostic to therapeutic colonoscopy. Endoscopy 2009;41: 941–51.
52. Jiminez-Perez J, Pastor G, Aznarez R, et al. Iatrogenic perforation in diagnostic colonoscopy related to the type of sedation [abstract]. Gastrointest Endosc 2000;51:AB3351.
53. Hansen JJ, Ulmer BJ, Rex DK. Technical performance of colonoscopy with nurse-administered propofol sedation. Am J Gastroenterol 2004;99:52–6.
54. Walker JA, McIntyre RD, Schleinitz PF, et al. Nurse-administered propofol sedation without anesthesia specialists in 9152 endoscopic cases in an ambulatory surgery center. Am J Gastroenterol 2003;98(8):1744–50.
55. Cohen LB, Weitman ES, Voynarovska M, et al. Gastroenterologist-directed propofol, midazolam and fentanyl for endoscopic sedation: adverse events during 4,213 procedures [abstract]. Gastrointest Endosc 2005;61:AB111.
56. Sharma VK, Nguyen CC, Crowell MD, et al. A national study of cardiopulmonary unplanned events after GI endoscopy. Gastrointest Endosc 2007;66(1):27–34.
57. Fu ES, Downs JB, Schweiger JW, et al. Supplemental oxygen impairs detection of hypoventilation by pulse oximetry. Chest 2004;126:1552–8.
58. Downs JB. Has oxygen administration delayed appropriate respiratory care? Fallacies regarding oxygen therapy. Respir Care 2003;48(6):611–20.
59. Qadeer MA, Vargo JJ, Khandwala F, et al. Propofol versus traditional sedative agents for gastrointestinal endoscopy: a meta-analysis. Clin Gastroenterol Hepatol 2005;3(11):1049–56.
60. Singh H, Poluha W, Cheung M, et al. Propofol for sedation during colonoscopy. Cochrane Database Syst Rev 2008;4:CD006268.

Management of High-Risk Colonoscopy Patients

Robert S. Bresalier, MD

KEYWORDS

- Colon cancer screening • Familial adenomatous polyposis
- Hereditary non-polyposis colorectal cancer
- Inflammatory bowel disease • Chromoendoscopy

Gastrointestinal (GI) malignancies account for more than 3 million new cancers per year worldwide and are responsible for almost 2.5 million deaths annually. Each year, approximately 1 million new cases of colorectal cancer (CRC) occur worldwide with substantial morbidity and mortality. For colon cancer in the United States, 147,000 new cases and 50,000 colon cancer–related deaths have been estimated for 2009.[1] The long natural history of colorectal neoplasia affords the opportunity to improve survival from this disease through preventive measures. Rapid growth of knowledge about the molecular and biologic characteristics of GI cancers has provided useful insights into the pathogenesis of GI neoplasms and cancer in general. Because most GI cancers arise over long periods as a result of interactions between genetic predisposition and environmental insults, it has become possible to identify preneoplastic and early neoplastic lesions better and to improve survival rates. Rapidly evolving knowledge of the pathogenesis and natural history of GI cancers, especially in high-risk groups, is allowing the development of new tools to identify those who will benefit most from preventive measures. Current, screening for adenomas, dysplasia, and early-stage invasive cancers provides the best opportunity to improve survival. Growing knowledge of CRC pathogenesis and its natural history is also allowing the better definition of proper surveilance intervals. Recently, guidelines for screening for colorectal neoplasia have been substantially revised by several organizations based on developing technologies and a growing body of data regarding the efficacy of CRC screening.[2–4] Although screening guidelines for the average-risk population provide a variety of options, screening of high-risk groups almost always includes colonoscopy. Proper risk stratification, understanding the natural history of each disease, and optimal techniques all help define quality colonoscopy in high-risk groups.

What defines a high-risk patient? Because the subject of this issue of *Gastrointestinal Endosocopy Clinics of North America* is "Quality Colonoscopy," this article deals principally with those individuals at high risk for developing CRC, although many

Department of Gastroenterology, Hepatology and Nutrition, The University of Texas M.D. Anderson Cancer Center, 1515 Holcombe Boulevard, Unit 1466, Houston, TX 77030-4009, USA
E-mail address: rbresali@mdanderson.org

Gastrointest Endoscopy Clin N Am 20 (2010) 629–640
doi:10.1016/j.giec.2010.07.015
1052-5157/10/$ – see front matter © 2010 Elsevier Inc. All rights reserved.

individuals included in this group also are at increased risk for developing other cancers in the GI tract and elsewhere. The term, *high-risk*, is a matter of interpretation, because the relative and absolute risks for colon cancer associated with some disease entities remain to be clearly defined. Value to society defined in terms of quality/cost and numbers of lives saved also differ from the magnitude of relative benefit in small, but very high-risk, groups (eg, familial adenomatous polypsosis). **Fig. 1** illustrates this point. Although the relative risk of CRC in a given population may be high, the total number of individuals in a particular high-risk group may be small. **Box 1** categorizes various groups according to risk based on current knowledge. Several recent reviews have provided guidelines for the clinical management of individuals at increased or high risk for developing CRC.[2,5–14] This review necessarily touches on overall screening and management but concentrates on the issues of quality colonoscopy.

MANAGEMENT OF INDIVIDUALS WITH THE LYNCH SYNDROME (HEREDITARY NONPOLYPOSIS COLORECTAL CANCER)

Lynch syndrome or HNPCC is the most common form of genetically determined colon cancer predisposition in which a specific genetic abnormality has been identified.[11,12] Lynch syndrome is an autosomal dominant disorder with high penetration and accounts for approximately 3% to 4% of CRCs. Approximately 80% of cases meeting the clinical criteria for Lynch syndrome are associated with germline mutations in genes responsible for repair of DNA errors, called mismatches, that occur during DNA replication. The majority of reported germline mutations in DNA mismatch repair (MMR) genes have been associated with the *MSH2* gene on chromosome 2 (40% to 50%) and the *MLH1* gene on chromosome 3 (20% to 30%). Mutations in *MSH6*, *PMS1*, and *PMS2* have also been reported. No locus has been identified, however, for many HNPCC families. The lifetime risk of CRC approaches 70% to 80% in affected individuals carrying a MMR gene mutation. During DNA synthesis, DNA polymerase may create single base-pair mismatches resulting in structural abnormalities (so-called loop-outs) involving unpaired bases. These alterations tend to occur at repetitive DNA sequences, termed *microsatellites*, leading to a microsatellite instability

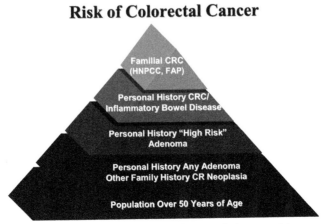

Risk of Colorectal Cancer

Familial CRC (HNPCC, FAP)

Personal History CRC/ Inflammatory Bowel Disease

Personal History "High Risk" Adenoma

Personal History Any Adenoma Other Family History CR Neoplasia

Population Over 50 Years of Age

Fig. 1. Relative risk of CRC in different groups. The top of the pyramid represents populations at highest risk but accounting for a relatively small proportion of CRC cases.

Box 1
Relative risk of developing colorectal cancer

Average risk

Individuals ≥50 years of age with

- No family history of colorectal neoplasia (adenoma or cancer)
- No personal history of adenoma or CRC
- No personal history of inflammatory bowel disease (IBD)

Increased risk

- Personal history of CRC
- Personal history of adenoma[a]
- Positive family history of sporadic CRC[b]
- Positive family history of sporadic adenoma[b]

High risk

- Hereditary nonpolyposis CRC (HNPCC) or Lynch syndrome
- Polyposis syndromes

  Classical familial adenomatous polyposis (FAP)

  Attenuated FAP

  MYH-associated polyposis

  Peutz-Jeghers syndrome

  Juvenile polyposis syndrome

  Hyperplastic polyposis syndrome

- IBD (ulcerative colitis [UC] or Crohn disease [CD])[c]

[a] The risk of developing CRC in individuals with a personal history of adenoma varies according to the size, histology, and multiplicity of index lesions.
[b] The risk of developing CRC in those with a positive family history of sporadic adenoma or CRC depends on the number and degree (first degree, second degree, and so forth) of affected relatives and the age at which neoplasia occurred in these individuals.
[c] Individuals with IBD have been categorized as "increased risk"[5] or "high risk"[2] according to different guidelines.

(MSI), a hallmark of CRC occurring in the setting of Lynch syndrome. The definition of HNPCC was standardized and most strictly defined by the International Collaborative Group on Hereditary Non-Polyposis Colorectal Cancer. These Amsterdam criteria include (1) at least three relatives with histologically verified CRC, one of them a first-degree relative of the other two (FAP excluded); (2) at least two successive generations affected; and (3) in one of the individuals, diagnosis of CRC before age 50 years. Because these criteria do not account for the frequent occurrence of extracolonic cancers in such families (endometrial, ovary, stomach, ureter/renal, pelvis, pancreas, brain, hepatobiliary tract, small bowel, and multiple sebaceous adenomas and carcinomas and keratoacanthomas in the Muir-Torre syndrome variant of Lynch syndrome) or for small kindreds, broader clinical criteria have been developed, including the modified Amsterdam criteria (Amsterdam II) and the revised Bethesda guidelines,[15] published by a National Cancer Institute–sponsored workshop on HNPCC (**Box 2**). The latter include CRC with MSI-H (presence of tumor-infiltrating

> **Box 2**
> **Amsterdam II and revised Bethesda guidelines for Lynch syndrome**
>
> *Amsterdam II criteria*
>
> There should be at least three relatives with CRC or with a Lynch syndrome–associated cancer (endometrium, small bowel, ureter, or renal pelvis).
>
> - One relative should be a first-degree relative of the other two
> - At least two successive generations should be affected
> - At least one tumor should be diagnosed before the age of 50 years
> - FAP should be excluded
> - Tumors should be verified by histologic examination
>
> *Revised Bethesda guidelines*
>
> - CRC diagnosed in an individual <50 years of age
> - Presence of synchronous or metachronous CRC or other Lynch syndrome–associated tumor[a] regardless of age
> - CRC with MSI-H phenotype diagnosed in an individual <60 years of age
> - Patient with CRC and a first-degree relative with a Lynch syndrome–related tumor, with one of the cancers diagnosed at <50 years of age
> - Patient with CRC with two or more first-degree or second-degree relatives with a Lynch syndrome–related tumor, regardless of age
>
> [a] Endometrial, ovary, stomach, ureter/renal, pelvis, pancreas, brain, hepatobiliary tract, small bowel, and multiple sebaceous adenomas and carcinomas and keratoacanthomas in the Muir-Torre syndrome variant of Lynch syndrome.

lymphocytes, Crohn-like lymphocytic reaction, mucinous/signet cell differentiation, or medullary growth pattern).

In Lynch syndrome, discrete polyps, but not polyposis, may antedate the cancers. Adenomas in the proximal colon may be flat or slightly raised lesions with foci of adenomatous change confined to the upper half of a crypt (flat adenomas). Lynch syndrome is characterized by a tendency toward proximal sites of colon tumors (approximately 70% of CRCs are proximal to the splenic flexure), multiple primary malignancies (synchronous and metachronous), and a higher incidence of mucinous carcinomas. These CRCs usually appear at age 40 to 50 years, 2 decades earlier than CRC in the general population.

Individuals with Lynch syndrome are at increased lifetime risk for developing CRC compared with the general population (70% to 80% vs 6%). Several studies suggest a higher CRC risk in men compared with women and a higher risk in *MLH1* mutation carriers than in *MSH2* mutation carriers. Development of metachronous primary CRCs is also common in Lynch syndrome, with one study reporting a risk of 40% for a second CRC within 7 years of the first cancer. Algorithmic approaches to screening and surveillance of families with Lynch syndrome or those suspected of having Lynch syndrome have been adopted by professional societies with clinical practice guidelines for genetic testing and risk assessment for patients and families.[2,5,16,17] Genetic testing and counseling is an essential part of quality care in families with known MMR gene mutations. Because 70% to 80% of CRCs in the setting of Lynch syndrome are proximal to the splenic flexure, colonoscopy is the mandated screening modality for the colon. Most guidelines suggest that screening begin at age 20 to 25 or 10 years before the youngest case in the immediate family and repeated every 1 to 2 years in at-risk individuals with MMR gene mutations (discussed later).

The evidence supporting colonoscopic surveillance in individuals with Lynch syndrome is provided by several observational studies.[18–24] A 15-year observational cohort study of HNPCC families from Finland demonstrated that in 133 at-risk individuals undergoing prospective asymptomatic screening at 3-year intervals, invasive CRC incidence was reduced by 62% compared with 119 controls from the same families who did not undergo surveillance.[18,19] Follow-up of these individuals demonstrated reduced mortality in those undergoing surveillance colonoscopy compared with those who did not undergo surveillance.[19] CRC occurred in 6% of screened individuals and 16% of unscreened individuals. These rates were 18% versus 41% in MMR carriers. All CRCs in the screened group were early stage with no associated mortality versus 9 deaths in the unscreened group. Several observational studies do show, however, that interval cancers develop within a 3-year interval after colonoscopy, and a study of 114 families with proved or suspected MMR mutations suggested that a surveillance interval of 2 years or less is required is required to diagnose CRC at an early stage in these individuals.[20] A recent study using the Dutch Lynch syndrome registry also concluded that members of Lynch syndrome families have a lower risk of developing CRC with surveillance interval of 1 to 2 years compared with interval of 2 to 3 years.[22] These observations and the evidence that there may be an accelerated rate of colon carcinogenesis in the setting of Lynch syndrome[11] have led to the recommendation that surveillance colonoscopy be performed every 1 to 2 years in at-risk individuals. Some have recommended, based on observational data concerning cumulative cancer rates, that the surveillance interval be reduced to 1 year after age 40.[11]

The success and cost-effectiveness of colon cancer screening and surveillance in any population is highly dependent on compliance with recommended guidelines. Quality colonoscopy requires that best practices regarding recommendations for screening and surveillance be adhered to by physicians and patients. This is not always the case. Stoffel and colleagues[25] conducted a study using a cross-sectional questionnaire among individuals with a personal or family history of CRC who fulfilled the Bethesda guidelines for evaluation of Lynch syndrome; 181 individuals further met the Amsterdam criteria for the Lynch syndrome and/or had an identified mutation in a MMR gene. Of these high-risk individuals, 73% had what was defined as an appropriate surveillance with colonoscopies every 2 years. Of those individuals who did not meet the criteria for a proper surveillance interval, 53% had colonoscopies at 3- to 5-year intervals. Because subjects were recruited through four US genetics clinics, compliance is likely to be worse in less specialized settings. As discussed previously, interval cancer does occur despite adherence to surveillance colonoscopy. It is also important to communicate to patients that despite surveillance, there is a small risk of developing CRC. In one recent study,[22] 6% of individuals developed CRC despite surveillance, and 10% of these cancers were at an advanced stage (Dukes C or stage III).

CRCs occurring in the setting of Lynch syndrome are often right sided and precursor adenomas are commonly flat.[11] This has led to the common use of red flag techniques, such as chromoendosocopy, in an attempt to better detect these lesions.

High-magnification colonoscopy with chromoendoscopy using indigo carmine or methylene blue may improve the detection of neoplastic lesions in the colon of individuals with Lynch syndrome.[26–29] Hurlstone and colleagues[26] performed back-to-back colonoscopies in 25 individuals who met the Amsterdam I criteria for HNPCC. Conventional colonoscopy with targeted chromoscopy was followed by pancolonic chromoscopic colonoscopy using indigo carmine. Panchromoscopy identified significantly more adenomas than conventional chromoscopy ($P = .001$) and a significantly higher number of flat adenomas ($P = .004$). In a small study, LeCompte and colleagues[27] found that indigo carmine dye spraying in the proximal colon increased adenoma detection. Stoffel and colleagues[28] evaluated the colonic adenoma miss rate among Lynch syndrome patients undergoing surveilance colonoscopy. The mean interval since last colonoscopy was 17.5 months. They compared the sensitivity of indigo carmine panchromoendoscopy with intensive white light inspection for identifying polyps missed by an initial standard colonoscopy performed during the same visit. Chromoendoscopy detected more polyps, but after controlling for several variables, chromoendosocopy did not detect more adenomas than intensive inspection in this pilot study of 28 individuals. This trial points out the importance of controlling for withdrawal times in such studies. There was an initial adenoma miss rate of 55% with the first white light screening colonoscopy. Additional adenomas were detected by both chromoendoscopy and intensive standard colonoscopy (20-minute pull back from cecum) on a second examination.

In approximately 30% of families that meet Amsterdam I criteria for Lynch syndrome, MSI testing and testing for MMR gemline mutations is negative.[29,30] These individuals develop CRC at a more advanced age and have fewer cancers than those with Lynch syndrome. In families without MMR deficiency, a less-intensive surveillance protocol is recommended with colonoscopy at 3- to 5-year intervals, starting at 5 to 10 years before the first diagnosis of CRC or at 45 years of age.[10]

Individuals in Lynch syndrome families who test negative for a known mutation and who are asymptomatic should undergo routine screening recommended for individuals with a family history of CRC.

MANAGEMENT OF INDIVIDUALS WITH FAMILIAL ADENOMATOUS POLYPOSIS

Classical FAP is characterized by the development of hundreds to thousands of adenomas in the colorectum as well as other extracolonic manifestations (including duodenal polyposis) and accounts for less than 1% of CRC. FAP is an autosomal dominant condition characterized by mutations in the *APC* gene located on chromosome 5q21. The lifetime risk of CRC in individuals with classic FAP is almost 100%, and CRC develops by a mean age of 40 to 50 years. The risk of developing CRC before age 20 is, however, low. In known FAP families, genetic testing is performed at adolescence to identify familial mutations. As with Lynch syndrome, quality assurance requires that such testing be accompanied by genetic counseling. Family members who test positive for an *APC* mutation should begin endosocopic surveillance from their early teens at yearly intervals.[5,10] Endosocopic surveillance should be lifelong due to the high penetrance of the disease. Because the rectum is affected in all cases, flexible sigmoidoscopy may be initially sufficient. If adenomas are detected, colonoscopy should be performed until colectomy is planned. If genetic testing is not done, flexible sigmoidoscopy or colonoscopy should be performed yearly between the ages of 10 to 15 and 24, every 2 years until age 34, every 3 years until age 44, and every 3 to 5 years thereafter.[5]

A variety of enhanced visualization techniques have been proposed to detect adenomas in at-risk individuals or after total abdominal colectomy with ileorectal anastomosis. One small study compared chromoendoscopy, narrow band imaging, and autofluorescence for detection of diminutive adenomas in individuals with FAP and intact colons. Colonoscopy with chromoendoscopy was superior to white light colonoscopy, autofluorescence imaging, and narrow band imaging for detection of diminutive adenomas.[31] Chromoendosocpy has been also shown to increase the detection of duodenal adenomas in individuals with FAP.[32]

Approximately 8% of families with FAP have an attenuated form characterized by fewer than 100 adenomas (average of 30), adenomas, cancers at an age older than classic FAP, and a frequent right-sided distribution of adenomas. Individuals in these families should undergo genetic testing for *APC* mutations, and affected individuals should begin colonoscopy at age 18 to 20 years. In individuals less than 21 years of age who have a small adenoma burden, colonoscopy and polypectomy should be performed every 1 to 2 years, but as with classical FAP, surgery should be performed in older individuals manifesting polyposis.

MANAGEMENT OF INDIVIDUALS WITH OTHER POLYPOSIS SYNDROMES

Biallelic mutation in the base excision repair gene *MUTYH* is associated with an autosomal recessive cancer susceptibility syndrome.[33,34] *MYH*-associated disease may manifest in a form similar to attenuated FAP (ie, polyposis), or with only a few adenomas. Adenomas are often serrated. The median age of presentation is in the mid-40s to late 50s. Colonoscopy surveillance of affected individuals should be performed every 1 to 2 years beginning at ages18 to 20.

A variety of hamartomatous polyposis syndromes are associated with an increased risk of CRC. Peutz-Jeghers syndrome is an autosomal dominant disease characterized by hamartomatous polyps of the small and large intestine and mucocutaneous pigmentation of the mouth, lips, nose, eyes, genitalia, or fingers. Extraintestinal cancers are common. The syndrome in most families has been mapped to the *STK11* serine threonine kinase 11 (*STK11*). Colonoscopy should be performed every 2 to 3 years beginning in the late teens.[5] Juvenile polyposis syndrome is characterized by at least three to five juvenile polyps of the colon, multiple juvenile polyps in the remainder of the GI tract, and a family history of juvenile polyposis. This is an autosomal dominant disease in which the cumulative risk for CRC may approach 40%. Germline mutations have been reported in *SMAD4* that encodes an intracellular mediator in the transforming growth factor β signaling pathway and bone morphogenetic protein receptor type 1A (*BMPR1A*). Colonoscopy should be performed beginning at age 15 in families with juvenile polyposis syndrome. Surveilance colonoscopy should be performed annually if polyps are found, and every 2 to 3 years if no polyps are found.[5]

MANAGMENT OF INDIVIDUALS WITH INFLAMMATORY BOWEL DISEASE

The risk of developing CRC is increased in individuals with UC and CD. The risk of CRC in individuals with IBD has been difficult to estimate in the past due to methodologic issues, but development of carcinoma is associated with cumulative risk over time. A large meta-analysis estimated the risk of cancer in patients with UC to be 2% after 10 years duration of disease, 8% after 20 years, and 18% after 30 years.[35] Data from the St Mark's Hospital 30-year surveillance program reported the cumulative risk of combined cancer and dysplasia to be 7.7% at 20 years and 15.8% at 30 years.[36] Several smaller recent studies have suggested lower risks. Despite a wide variation of reported risk for CRC in CD, recent data have led to a consensus that the risk in both UC and CD is similar.[14] The risk for development of CRC in IBD is higher in those with longer disease duration, more extensive colitis (macroscopic or microscopic), primary sclerosing cholangitis (UC), and positive family history of sporadic CRC. Indirect evidence suggests that the severity of endoscopic and histologic inflammation is associated with progression to CRC, but studies have not been definitive. Dysplasia defined as an unequivocal neoplastic epithelium confined to the basement membrane (ie, intraepithelial neoplasia) is the best and most reliable marker of risk for CRC in IBD.[13,14] It is the search for dysplasia that forms the basis for colonoscopic surveillance in individuals with IBD.

In the colon, dysplasia is characterized by a combination of microscopic crypt alterations and cytologic atypia.[37,38] The more pronounced these changes, the higher the degree of dysplasia. Dysplasia is present in more than 90% of colons in which UC is associated with carcinoma,[16] and the evidence is compelling that dysplasia represents a precursor to adenocarcinoma. The assumption that colon carcinogenesis in the setting of IBD follows a sequential progression from low-grade dysplasia to high-grade dysplasia to invasive carcinoma forms the basis for screening and surveillance in the setting of IBD, but this sequence of progression may not be absolute. Dysplasia may occur in flat mucosa or in the form of elevated lesions so-called dysplasia-associated mass lesions. Current evidence suggests with a high degree of certainty that patients with IBD and non–adenoma-like dysplasia occurring in raised lesions should undergo colectomy and that colectomy for flat high-grade dysplasia treats undiagnosed synchronous cancers and prevents the occurrence of future cancers. Because the interepretation of the grade of dysplasia determines clinical management (**Fig. 2**), an important quality issue is the correct histologic intereptetation of dysplasia. This is an important issue because the overall level of agreement even among expert pathologists has been shown in clinical trials to be only fair. Maximizing the value of the endosocopist-pathologist partnership is, therefore, essential (see the article by Snover elsewhere in this issue for further exploration of this topic).

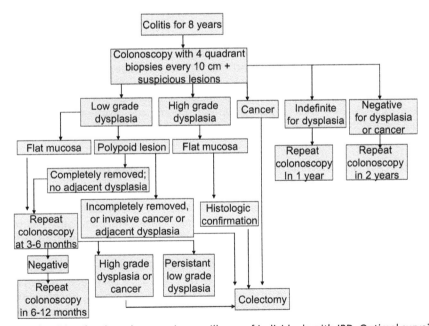

Fig. 2. Algorithm for the colonoscopic surveillance of individuals with IBD. Optimal surveillance intervals have not been clearly defined. Recommendations are based on existing data. Recommendations are for individuals with UC and Crohn colitis. Pancolonic dye spraying chromoendoscopy with targeted biopsies of abnormal areas has been recommended by several guidelines.

Surveillance colonoscopy in patients with IBD is commonly performed based on the assumption that identification of intraepithelial neoplasia (ie, dysplasia) and early invasive carcinoma improves survival. Although randomized controlled trials have not been performed to prove that surveillance colonoscopy in this setting improves survival, many case-controlled trials suggest that surveillance is likely to be effective (and cost effective) at reducing the risk of death from IBD-associated cancer.[39] Quality issues that influence the success of surveillance colonoscopy include endoscopic recognition of dysplasia; endoscopic resectability and completeness of resection of adenoma-like polypoid lesions; adequacy of mucosal sampling; the ability to recognize and navigate anatomic factors, such as strictures and inflammatory pseudopolyps, which may interfere with sampling and the ability to detect dysplasia; and patient acceptance and compliance.[14]

Much like the case of screening and surveillance of average-risk and other high-risk individuals (see the article by Hewett and Rex elsewhere in this issue for further exploration of this topic), the success of surveillance colonoscopy in the setting of IBD depends on the knowledge, expertise, and care of the endoscopist performing the procedure. Although dysplasia commonly occurs in flat mucosa, mucosal changes suggesting dysplasia in IBD may often be recognized by an experienced endosocopist.[40] Most recommendations[14,41,42] specify that screening colonoscopy in patients with UC and CD be performed to rule out neoplasia beginning 8 to 10 years after onset of symptoms. Subsequent surveillance intervals may depend on clinical risk factors. The American Gastroenterological Association (AGA) Institute technical review panel suggests that patients with extensive or left-sided colitis begin surveillance 1 to 2 years after initial screening endoscopy and then, after two negative examinations, every 1 to 3 years.[14] Ideally, surveillance should be performed during periods of remission. Patients with primary sclerosing cholangitis should begin surveillance at the time of diagnosis and yearly thereafter. Patients with active inflammation; anatomic abnormalities, such as strictures and multiple inflammatory pseudopolyps; and a history of CRC in first-degree relatives may benefit from more frequent surveillance intervals.

Cleansing of the bowel should be optimal to maximize visualization of the entire mucosa. The success of surveillance depends on the adequacy of mucosal sampling. A study by Rubin and colleagues[43] indicated that 33 and 64 biopsy specimens were required to detect dysplasia with 90% and 95% probabilities, respectively, a standard adhered to by few practicing gastroenterologists. Four-quadrant biopsies should be taken from approximately every 10 cm of colon, and specimens from each anatomic segment should be submitted separately to avoid confusion as to the location of dysplasia, if detected. Recommendations from the Crohn's and Colitis Foundation of America,[41] the British Society of Gastroenterology, and the AGA Institute all include the use of chromoendoscopy with pancolonic dye spraying and targeted biopsies of abnormal areas. Several studies have suggested that use of this technique may be more effective than routine endoscopy with multiple non-targeted biopsies.[45–47] A recent US study examined 115 individuals with IBD at high risk for dysplasia.[47] Colonoscopies included random 4-quadrant biopsies every 10 cm, targeted biopsies of suspicious lesions detected without chromoendoscopy, and targeted biopsies of lesions detected by chromoendoscopy. Chromoendoscopy-targeted biopsies led to the detection of significantly more individuals with dysplasia (mostly low grade) compared with random biopsies or other targeted biopsies. The use of other red flag techniques, such as narrow band imaging, fluorescence endoscopy, optical coherence tomography, and confocal endomicroscopy, have been studied as adjunctive techniques in small groups of patients with IBD. Kiesslich and colleagues[45] randomized 161 patients with UC in remission to conventional white light colonoscopy or panchromoendosocopy plus endomicroscopy-targeted biopsies to detect dysplasia or CRC. Chromoendoscopy plus endomicroscopy detected 4.75-fold more neoplastic lesions ($P = .005$) compared with conventional colonoscopy. Analysis of the data also suggested that use of enhanced imaging techniques leads to the need for substantially fewer biopsies than random biopsies taken at standard colonoscopy.

The success and cost-effectiveness of colon cancer screening and surveillance in general is highly dependent on patient and physician compliance. This is also true of surveillance in the setting of IBD. More frequent physician visits were associated with a decreased risk of developing CRC (odds ratio 0.16; 95% CI, 0.04–0.60) in patients with UC in a case-control study that compared 102 cases of CRC in UC with matched controls.[48]

REFERENCES

1. Jemal A, Siegal R, Ward E, et al. Cancer statistics, 2009. CA Cancer J Clin 2009; 59:225–49.
2. Levin B, Lieberman DA, Mcfarland B, et al. Screening and surveillance for the early detection of colorectal cancer and adenomatous polyps, 2008: a joint guideline from the American Cancer Society, the US Multi-Society Task Force on Colorectal Cancer, and the American College of Radiology. CA Cancer J Clin 2008;58:130–60.
3. U.S. Preventative Services Task Force. Screening for Colorectal Cancer: U.S. Preventative services task force recommendation statement. Ann Intern Med 2008;149:627–37.
4. Rex DK, Johnson DA, Anderson JC, et al. American college of gastroenterology guidelines for colorectal cancer screening 2008. Am J Gastroenterol 2009;104: 739–50.
5. Burt RW, Barthel JS, Dunn KB, et al. NCCN clinical practice guidelines in oncology. Colorectal cancer screening. J Natl Compr Canc Netw 2010;8:8–61.
6. Sung JJ, Lau JW, Young GP, et al. Asia Pacific consensus recommendations for colorectal cancer screening. Gut 2008;57:1166–76.
7. Bresalier RS. Early detection of and screening for colorectal cancer. Gut Liver 2009;3:69–80.
8. Rex DK, Kahi CJ, Levin B, et al. Guidelines for colonoscopy surveillance after cancer resection: a consensus update by the American cancer Society and the US Multi-society task force on colorectal cancer. Gastroenterology 2006;130: 1865–71.
9. Winawer SJ, Zauber AG, Fletcher RH, et al. Guidelines for colonoscopy surveillance after polypectomy: a consensus update by the US Multi-Society Task Force on Colorectal cancer and the American Cancer Society. Gastroenterology 2006; 130:1872–85.
10. Vasen HF, Moslein G, Alonso A, et al. Guidelines for the clinical management of familial adenomatous polyposis (FAP). Gut 2008;57:704–13.
11. Lynch HT, Lynch PM, Lanspa SJ, et al. Review of the Lynch syndrome:history, molecular genetics, screening, differential diagnosis, and medicolegal ramifications. Clin Genet 2009;76:1–18.
12. Grover S, Syngal S. Risk assessment, genetic testing, and management of lynch syndrome. J Natl Compr Canc Netw 2010;8:98–106.
13. Potack J, Itzkowitz SH. Colorectal cancer in inflammatory bowel disease. Gut Liver 2008;2:61–73.

14. Farraye FA, Odze RD, Eaden J, et al. AGA technical review on the diagnosis and management of colorectal neoplasia in inflammatory bowel disease. Gastroenterology 2010;138:746–74.

15. Umar A, Boland CR, Terdiman JP, et al. Revised bethesda guidelines for herditary nonpolyposis colorectal cancer (lynch syndrome) and microstellite instability. J Natl Cancer Inst 2004;96:261–8.

16. Church J, Simmang C, Standards Task Force American Society of Colon and Rectal Surgeons, et al. Practice parameters for the treatment of patients with dominantly inherited colorectal cancer (familial polyposis, hereditary nonpolyposis colorectal cancer). Dis Colon Rectum 2003;46:1001–12.

17. Lindor NM, Peterson GM, Hadley DW, et al. Recommendations for the care of individuals with an inherited predisposition to Lynch syndrome:a systematic review. JAMA 2006;296:1507–17.

18. Jarvinen HJ, Mecklin JP, Sistonen P. Screening reduces colorectal cancer rate in families with hereditary nonpolyposis colorectal cancer. Gastroenterology 1995; 108:1405–11.

19. Jarvinen HJ, Aarnio M, Mustonen H, et al. Controlled 15-year trial on screening for colorectal cancer in families with hereditary nonpolyposis colorectal cancer. Gastroenterology 2000;118:829–34.

20. de Vos tot Neverveen Cappel WH, Nagengast FM, Griffioen G, et al. Surveillance for hereditary nonpolyposis colorectal cancer. Dis Colon Rectum 2002;45: 1588–94.

21. Dove-Edwin I, Sasieni P, Adams J, et al. Prevention of colorectal cancer by colonoscopic surveillance in individuals with a family history of colorectal cancer. BMJ 2005;331:1047.

22. Vasen HF, Abdirahman M, Brohet R, et al. 1–2 year surveilance intervals reduce risk of colorectal cancer in families with Lynch syndrome. Gastroenterology 2010; 138:2300–6.

23. Vasen HF, Moslein G, Alonso A, et al. Guidelines for the clinical management of Lynch syndrome (hereditary non-polypsosis cancer). J Med Genet 2007;44: 353–62.

24. de Jong AE, Hendricks YM, Kleibuker JH, et al. Shift in mortality due to due to surveillance in the Lynch syndrome. Gastroenterology 2006;130:665–71.

25. Stoffel EM, Mercado RC, Kohlmann W, et al. Prevalence and predictors of appropriate colorectal cancer surveillance in Lynch syndrome. Am J Gastroenterol 2010;105:1851–60.

26. Hurlsone DP, Karajeh M, Cross SS. The role of magnification-chromoscopic colonoscopy in hereditary nonpolyposis colorectal cancer screening: a prospective back-to-back endosocpy study. Am J Gastroenterol 2005;100:2167–73.

27. LeCompte T, Cellier C, Meatchi T, et al. Chromoendosocpic colonoscopy for detecting preneoplastic lesions in hereditary nonpolyposis colorectal cancer. Clin Gastroenterol Hepatol 2005;3:897–902.

28. Stoffel EM, Turgeon DK, Stockwell DH, et al. Missed adenomas during colonoscopic surveillance in individuals with Lynch syndrome (hereditary nonpoyposis colorectal cancer). Cancer Prev Res 2008;1:470–5.

29. Lindor NM, Rabe K, Peterson GM, et al. Lower cancer incidence in Amsterdam-I criteria families without mismatch repair deficiency. Familial colorectal cancer type X. JAMA 2005;293:1979–85.

30. Llor X, Pons E, Xicola RE, et al. Differential features of colorectal cancers fulfilling Amsterdam criteria without involvement of the mutator pathway. Clin cancer Res 2005;11:7304–10.

31. Matsumoto T, Fujisawa R, Nakamura R, et al. Chromoendoscopy, narrow band imaging colonoscopy, and autofluorescence colonoscopy for detection of diminutive colorectal neoplasia in familial adenomatous polyposis. Dis Colon Rectum 2009;52:1160–5.

32. Dekker E, Boparai KS, Poley JW, et al. High resolution endosocopy and the additional value of chromoendosocopy in the evaluation of duodenal adenomatosis in patients with familial adenomatous polyposis. Endoscopy 2009;41:666–9.

33. Al-Tassen N, Chmiel NH, Maynard J, et al. Inherited variants of MYH associated with somatic G: C-T: a mutations in colorectal tumors. Nat Genet 2002;30:227–32.

34. Vogt S, Jones N, Christian D, et al. Expanded extracolonic tumor spectrum in MUTYH-associated polyposis. Gastroenterology 2009;137:1976–85.

35. Eaden JA, Abrams KR, Mayberry JF. The risk of colorectal cancer in ulcerative colitis, a meta-analysis. Gut 2001;48:526–35.

36. Rutter MD, Saunders BP, Wilkinson KH, et al. Thirty-year analysis of a colonoscopic surveillance program for neoplasia in ulcerative colitis. Gastroenterology 2006;130:1030–8.

37. Riddell RH, Goldman H, Ransohoff DF, et al. Dysplasia in inflammatory bowel disease:standardized classification with provisional clinical applications. Hum Pathol 1983;14:931–68.

38. Schlemper RJ, Riddell RH, Kato Y, et al. The Vienna classification of gastrointestinal epithelial neoplasia. Gut 2000;47:251–5.

39. Mpofu C, Watson AJ, Rhodes JM. Strategies for detecting colon cancer and/or dysplasia in patients with inflammatory bowel disease. Cochrane Database Syst Rev 2004;2:CD000279.

40. Rutter MD, Saunders BP, Wilkinson KH, et al. Most dysplasia in ulcerative colitis is visible at colonoscopy. Gastrointest Endosc 2004;60:334–9.

41. Itzkowitz SH, Present DH. Consensus conference:colorectal cancer screening and surveillance in inflammatory bowel disease. Inflamm Bowel Dis 2005;11: 314–21.

42. Carter MJ, Lobo AJ, Travis SP. Guidelines for the management of inflammatory bowel disease in adults. Gut 2004;53(Suppl 5):V1–16.

43. Rubin CE, Haggit RC, Burmer GC, et al. DNA aneuploidy in colonic biopsies predicts future development of dysplasia in ulcerative coloitis. Gastroenterology 1992;103:1611–20.

44. Marion JF, Waye JD, Present DH, et al. Chromoendoscopy-targeted biopsies are superior to standard colonoscopic surveillance for detecting dysplasia in inflammatory bowel disease patients: a prospective endosocopic trial. Am J Gastroenterol 2008;103:2342–9.

45. Kiesslich R, Goetz M, Lammersdorf K, et al. Chromoendoscopy-guided endomicroscopy increases the diagnostic yield of intraepithelial neoplasia in ulcerative colitis. Gastroenterol 2007;132:874–82.

46. Hurlstone DP, Sanders DS, Lobo AJ, et al. Indigo carmine-assisted high-magnification chromoscopic colonoscopy for the detection and characterisation of intraepithelial dysplasia in inflammatory bowel disease: a prospective evaluation. Endoscopy 2005;37:1186–92.

47. Li CQ, Xie XJ, Yu T, et al. Classification of inflammation activity in ulcerative colitis by confocal lasar endomicroscopy. Am J Gastroenterol 2010;105:1391–6.

48. Eaden J, Abrams K, Ekbom A, et al. Colonoscopic cancer prevention in ulcerative colitis:a case-control study. Aliment Pharmacol Ther 2004;19:145–53.

Maximizing the Value of the Endoscopist–Pathologist Partnership in the Management of Colorectal Polyps and Carcinoma

Dale C. Snover, MD

KEYWORDS

- Pathology • Polyps • Adenocarcinoma • Adenoma
- Serrated adenoma • Microsatellite instability

Good communication between clinician and pathologist is essential for optimal patient care and management of colorectal polyps and carcinoma. General principles of communication include making sure that the pathologist as well as the endoscopist has all the information needed to make an accurate diagnosis and that the pathologist communicate the diagnosis back to the endoscopist in a clear and timely fashion. In recent years, the increasing complexity of the classification of colorectal polyps and carcinomas has added to the need for clear communication pathways between clinician and pathologist. The first part of this article is devoted to a brief outline of general communication issues; the second is discussion of current concepts in colorectal polyps and carcinomas.

Communication begins with, but should not be restricted to, the pathology requisition form that should always list the source of the specimen, including the specific location in the colon, the clinical differential diagnosis, and any special requests. A description of the endoscopic findings and procedure (eg, biopsy vs polypectomy) as well as the outcome of the procedure (ie, complete vs incomplete excision of a lesion) is essential and is easily accomplished by sending a copy of the endoscopy report to pathology with the specimen. If there are findings that an endoscopist specifically wants to have addressed, this should be stated on the requisition. Family history

---

Department of Pathology, Fairview Southdale Hospital, 6401 France Avenue South, Edina, MN 55435, USA
E-mail address: snoverd@umn.edu

Gastrointest Endoscopy Clin N Am 20 (2010) 641–657
doi:10.1016/j.giec.2010.07.004
1052-5157/10/$ – see front matter © 2010 Elsevier Inc. All rights reserved.

giendo.theclinics.com

may be relevant in cases of colorectal polyps or carcinomas, in particular if there is a possibility of Lynch syndrome for which additional work-up of the carcinoma for absence of mismatch repair (MMR) enzymes may be useful for deciding on proper therapy of the lesion (discussed later).

All pathology reports should specifically mention the site of the biopsy. If a specific site is not submitted with the specimen, that should be stated in the report. There should be a gross description of the specimen that includes, for biopsy specimens, the number and approximate size of fragments in the container and, for polypectomy specimens, a specific description indicating if the polyp was intact or fragmented and, if fragmented, how many fragments were present. If multiple polyps are submitted in one container, they should be handled individually by submitting in separate blocks for processing or by inking the different polyp fragments different colors. If a resection line of a polyp can be grossly identified, the margin should be inked and the polyp sectioned through that margin. In some cases, with a large number of biopsy fragments, an accurate count may not be possible but an estimate should be made. One importance of fragment counts, particularly if how many biopsies were taken is stated in the endoscopy report, is that it allows confirmation that all of the submitted tissue was included in the block and slide and that no tissue was lost. Alternatively, occasionally there are more pieces of tissue on the slide than were counted in the container. This most often occurs because tissue fragments stick together in the container and are miscounted as one when there are really two fragments present, but occasionally this indicates tissue cross-contamination from another patient's material. This becomes important if one of the fragments shows disparate histologic features. In laboratories processing many different types of tissue, the contaminating tissue likely is of a different organ than the gastrointestinal (GI) tract and is readily identifiable as not belonging to the case; however, in laboratories processing only GI cases, such easy identification is often not possible. This can lead to potentially disastrous consequences. I have seen cases of cross-contamination of malignant tissue into a GI biopsy that is otherwise benign, potentially leading to misdiagnosis and unnecessary surgery. Although it is impossible to prevent all cross-contamination, proper procedure in the pathology laboratory should make this rare. Cross-contamination is a situation, however, in which proper communication can be helpful. Oftentimes in these cases, the worrisome findings are present in only one of multiple biopsies and seem out of context if the pathologist knows the clinical situation and endoscopic findings. The mistaken findings may not correlate with the endoscopic findings. In cases where there seems to be a discrepancy between the clinical findings and the results of the biopsy, careful attention to number of fragments and rapid communication between clinician and pathologist may prevent an unfortunate outcome.

Other essential elements of the pathology report should include a statement of adequacy of the biopsy, a diagnosis, and recommendations for further evaluation in cases of nondiagnostic specimens for which the pathologist thinks that the biopsy may not be adequate. Biopsy of a mass lesion that consists only of superficial ulcer debris, for example, may lead to a suggestion for rebiopsy if the index of suspicion for malignancy is high. In cases of neoplastic colorectal polyps, the report should include a specific diagnosis, including elements considered indicative of advanced neoplasia and if the polyp contains a carcinoma; then, if possible, there should be a statement regarding adequacy of excision of the lesion based on risk factors (described later). In many cases of polypectomy, a statement regarding adequacy of excision cannot be made because the polyp is removed in a piecemeal fashion or because of suboptimal orientation of the specimen. Therefore, for most adenomas without malignancy, adequacy of excision is best determined by an endoscopist. Essential elements of a pathology report for a polyp or carcinoma specimen are summarized in **Box 1**.

Ideally all pathology departments should have a critical diagnosis call list (ie, a list of diagnoses for which the responsible clinician should be called with the diagnosis) rather than just relying on the pathology report to convey the results. This list typically includes conditions requiring immediate clinical attention (for example, opportunistic infections in immunocompromsed patients), conditions requiring rapid follow-up, or conditions that might not be expected based on the clinical history or endoscopic findings. For example, the finding of carcinoma in a biopsy taken from a small erosion that was not considered suspicious for carcinoma, is best discussed directly with an endoscopist, as are carcinomas arising in polypectomy specimens. The critical diagnosis list cannot be standardized for all laboratories but is best developed jointly between the gastroenterologist and pathologist because there are some things that certain gastroenterologists might want immediate notification of whereas others might not. If a critical diagnosis call list is developed, it is crucial for all pathologists in the servicing pathology group to always abide by the list, because with such a list, the presumption is that these diagnoses will be called, and if they are not, there may well be a presumption that all is fine. A typical critical diagnosis call list is shown in **Box 2**.

Turnaround time for diagnosis is important to patient management; however, speed of diagnosis should never take precedence over accuracy. It is reasonable to expect all biopsies to be examined by a pathologist within 1 working day of accessioning of the specimen in the pathology laboratory, with a written report available within 1 to 2 days unless there are extenuating circumstances (need for additional tissue levels or

---

Box 1

Items to be included in pathology reports for colorectal polyp and carcinoma biopsy/polypectomy specimens

A gross description, including confirmation of the labeling of the specimen along with a count of the number of tissue pieces in the container

A specific location of each part of the specimen (or a statement, "site not specified," if no location was provided with the specimen)

A specific procedure for each part of the specimen (ie, biopsy vs polypectomy)

A specific diagnosis for each part of the specimen

If a specimen is inadequate for diagnosis, a statement to that effect with an explanation of why the specimen is inadequate

For conventional adenoma and traditional serrated adenoma (TSA), a specific statement regarding the absence or presence of high-grade dysplasia or invasive malignancy

For sessile serrated adenoma (SSA), a specific statement regarding absence or presence of cytologic dysplasia or malignancy

For any adenoma, a statement regarding adequacy of excision (completely excised, incompletely excised, or cannot determine due to the nature of the specimen [eg, piecemeal resection])

For adenoma with invasive carcinoma, statements regarding adequacy of excision, grade of the carcinoma (low vs high grade), and presence or absence of lymphovascular invasion.

For invasive carcinoma, a statement regarding absence or presence of features of microsatellite instability (or "cannot determine because of small sampling")

Box 2
Typical critical diagnosis call list for colonoscopic specimens

All malignancies

SSA with cytologic dysplasia

Dysplasia in Barrett esophagus or inflammatory bowel disease

Unusual/opportunistic infections (excluding Helicobacter and Candida; including cytomegalovirus and herpes)

Pseudomembranous colitis but only if it is not a suspicion in the endoscopy report or requisition (this is to cover unexpected community acquired pseudomembranous colitis)

---

special stains, for example). In cases for which there is expected to be a delay in diagnosis, for example, cases sent for a consultation opinion, the clinician should be called and informed of the delay (with an explanation of the issue requiring consultation or delay). All cases fitting the critical diagnosis category should be called to the responsible clinician on the day of diagnosis (1 day after receipt of the biopsy). It is the responsibility of the clinician to assure notification the patient of the diagnosis in a timely fashion as well, typically within 2 to 3 days of receiving the diagnosis. Total time from biopsy to notification of the patient typically is 5 to 7 working days, depending somewhat on the peculiarities of the specific practice. If specimens need to be shipped to a laboratory, that may add a day, and any time required to send paper reports to offices also lead to delay. Regardless of these issues, expectations should be set by the office and conveyed to the patient at the time of biopsy, and fulfillment of these expectations should be monitored to avoid having patients slip through the cracks. Unnecessary delays at any point in the process (eg, delays in calling a patient because the clinician is on vacation or delays caused by lost reports not noted by a monitoring system) are inappropriate under any circumstance.

The remainder of this article is devoted to current concepts in the pathology of colorectal neoplasia with emphasis on new developments and communication issues.

CURRENT CONCEPTS OF THE PATHOLOGY OF COLON POLYPS AND CANCERS

From the time of the discovery of the APC mutation and the development of the Fearon-Vogelstein model of the suppressor pathway to colorectal carcinoma in 1990 until the late 1990s, when the alternative mutator pathway was discovered, essentially all colorectal carcinoma was thought to arise along the suppressor pathway.[1] Carcinoma arising via the suppressor pathway is now known as CpG island methylated phenotype negative, microsatellite stable (CIMP−, MSS) carcinoma (CIMP and MSS are discussed later). The precursor lesion for this type of carcinoma as well as for CIMP−, microsatellite instable (CIMP−, MSI) carcinoma occurring in Lynch syndrome along the mutator pathway is the conventional adenoma (the term, *conventional adenoma*, is used to distinguish adenomas with APC mutations from the new category of *serrated adenomas*, described later). Essentially all screening and intervention trials are focused on removal or prevention of conventional adenomas. As few as 65% of colorectal carcinoma may arise from conventional adenomas, however, with the remaining 35% probably developing from SSAs (15% occurring as sporadic MSI carcinomas (CIMP+, MSI) and 20% as CIMP+, MSS carcinoma.[2]

The term, *CIMP+*, refers to lesions having large numbers of genes that are silenced by methylation (rather than mutation) of cytosine to guanine nucleotide pairs, referred to as CpG islands, in their promoter regions. If the methylation occurs at the MLH1 gene, the tumors lose their ability to repair mutations resulting from mismatching of nucleotide pairs during DNA replication (MLH1 is one of the MMR genes), which leads to variation of the size of microsatellite regions within the cell's DNA; this variation in size is referred to as MSI (testing for MSI is discussed later); MSI refers to a high degree of MSI as opposed to tumors with no or a low degree of MSI, which are usually combined as MSS tumors). This same MSI phenomenon occurs in Lynch syndrome but the mechanism is a germline mutation in one of the MMR genes rather than methylation, and the tumors are CIMP−. The net effect of this loss of MMR is that spontaneous mutations that occur in cells are not repaired, leading to the development of carcinoma (with the increased rate of mutations leading to the designation mutator pathway). Tumors that do not demonstrate microsatellite instability are designated MSS. The specific molecular pathway of the CIMP+, MSS group has not been well characterized to date; the specific genes involved with carcinogenesis in this group are unknown.

SSAs are CIMP+ adenomas that start out with BRAF rather than APC mutations, and CIMP+ carcinomas arise in SSAs (discussed later); the designation, serrated pathway, is used for this pathway.[3,4] Serrated pathway is not a synonym for the mutator pathway, however, because not all tumors with MSI arise in SSAs (carcinoma in Lynch syndrome arises from conventional adenoma not from SSA), and not all tumors arising from SSAs are MSI (ie, the CIMP+, MSS group). The fact that until the last few years SSAs were usually diagnosed as hyperplastic polyps (HPs) and ignored as a potentially preneoplastic lesion may account for screening programs having been more successful in decreasing the rate of left-sided colorectal carcinoma versus right-sided cancers, because SSAs and CIMP+ carcinomas occur predominantly in the right colon.[5,6] In addition, it is likely that cancers arising in SSAs account for a significant percentage of interval carcinomas seen in screening programs, because of failure to recognize and remove SSAs and because some SSAs become malignant while small (discussed later). Interval cancers are disproportionately CIMP+, MSI and CIMP+, MSS, supporting this contention.[7,8] The various recognized pathways to colorectal carcinoma are summarized in **Table 1**.

The recognition of this new family of serrated polyps has changed the classification scheme of benign polyps of the large intestine. A current scheme is shown in **Box 3**.

CONVENTIONAL ADENOMAS (CIMP−, PREDOMINANTLY APC MUTATED)

The pathology of conventional adenomas is well known to all pathologists. The key feature is the presence of immature cytologically dysplastic cells creating a polyp. These cells usually have elongated hyperchromatic pseudostratified nuclei and demonstrate abundant mitotic activity (**Fig. 1**). Before the recognition of SSA, the presence of this cytologic dysplasia was used as a defining feature for premalignant lesions of the large intestine (adenomas), although this is now known not to be the case for SSA; hence, dysplasia need not be a prerequisite for the diagnosis of adenoma.

Conventional adenomas are subclassified based on the presence and extent of formation of villi or finger-like projections. Villi are associated with a greater risk for the development of carcinoma and with an increased rate of metachronous recurrence of polyps; hence, villiform lesions are designated as one type of advanced adenoma.[9,10] Typically, lesions are classified as tubular adenomas if less than 25% of the surface area is villous, tubulovillous adenomas if between 25% and 75% is villous, and villous adenomas if greater than 75% is villous (**Fig. 2**) (if the proper prefix [eg, tubulovillous] is used for a conventional adenoma, then the term *conventional* is

Table 1
Pathways to colorectal carcinoma

Pathway	Precursor Lesion	Initiating Mutation	Promoting Abnormalities	Type of Carcinoma	Percentage of all Carcinomas
Suppressor	Conventional adenoma	APC gene	Additional mutations to Kras, p53, etc.	CIMP−, MSS	60%
Lynch syndrome mutator	Conventional adenoma	MMR gene (MSH2, MLH1, MSH6, PMS2)	Unrepaired mutations of other critical genes (currently unknown)	CIMP−, MSI	5%
Sporadic mutator	SSA	BRAF	Methylation of MLH1 gene followed by unrepaired mutations of other critical genes (currently unknown)	CIMP+, MSI	15%
CIMP+, MSS pathway	SSA	BRAF	Methylation of unknown genes promoting development of cancer	CIMP+, MSS	20%

Box 3
Current classification of epithelial colorectal polyps

Neoplastic polyps

    Conventional adenomas (tubular, tubulovillous, and villous)

    SSA[a]

    SSA[a] with cytologic dysplasia

    TSA[b]

HP

    Microvesicular HP[c]

    Goblet cell–rich HP[c]

    Mucin-poor HP[c]

Hamartomatous polyps (Peutz-Jeghers, retention [juvenile], and Cowden type)

    Peutz-Jeghers polyp

    Cowden-type polyp

    Juvenile (retention) polyp

[a] The term, *sessile serrated polyp (SSP)*, is preferred by some authors and is an acceptable synonym for SSA at the current time.
[b] The term, *serrated adenoma*, without a qualifier (ie, traditional) is not considered acceptable and may be confusing.
[c] Use of the subtypes of HPs is optional at the current time.

---

not needed for diagnosis). Some investigators have challenged the reproducibility and clinical significance of villous architecture, arguing that size is a better indicator of advanced lesions, although in some studies villi were a more powerful predictor of recurrent adenomas than size.[11–13] It is the recommended standard to report conventional adenomas using this classification. Any lesion more than 25% villous is considered an advanced lesion for follow-up purposes.

The development of carcinoma in conventional adenomas is a stepwise process with increasing degrees of dysplasia, which correspond to accumulation of multiple mutations over time. A majority of conventional adenomas seem never to become malignant and it has been estimated that in a general risk population, 100 conventional

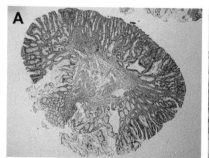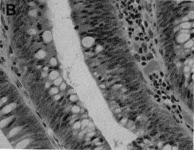

Fig. 1. Tubular adenoma. (*A*) Tubular adenomas demonstrate dysplasic changes starting at the tops of the crypts and extending downward, creating a dome-shaped or pedunculated polyp. (*B*) Conventional adenomas of all types are characterized by cytologically dysplastic cells with abundant mitotic activity.

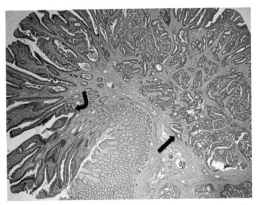

Fig. 2. Villous adenoma with adenocarcinoma. This lesion shows long finger-like projections (*curved arrow*) characteristic of villous architecture. In this case there is an associated low-grade adenocarcinoma in the right of the photo (*straight arrow*).

adenomas have to be removed to prevent a single carcinoma. The ratio of adenomas to carcinomas in the general risk population seems to be more than 10 to 1. In Lynch syndrome, however, progression seems more likely, no doubt because of the absence of mutation repair, and there is almost a 1-to-1 ratio of adenomas to carcinomas.[14] Morphologically the most advanced stage of progression before the actual development of invasive carcinoma is high-grade dysplasia (HGD). HGD can be diagnosed on the basis of cytologic or architectural changes (**Fig. 3**). The most common characteristic of HGD is cribriform architecture with gland-in-gland formation, distinguishable from carcinoma only by the lack of invasion below the muscularis mucosae. The reproducibility of HGD is probably less than that of villiform architecture, although this has been difficult to study because of its low incidence and because there is no gold standard that proves that one pathologist's idea of HGD has more meaning than another's. Therefore, some investigators have argued that reporting of HGD is meaningless, and a recent meta-analysis failed to show an association of HGD with metachronous adenomas.[15] Nevertheless, as with villous architecture, the standard of practice in recommended guidelines at the current time is to report HGD as a second type of advanced adenoma. Although HGD may not indicate high risk of polyp recurrence, because HGD is the immediate precursor to invasive carcinoma, if a lesion with

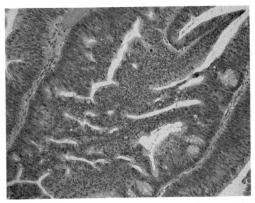

Fig. 3. HGD from the lesion in **Fig. 2**, with a complex cribriform architecture.

HGD is not completely resected it is always possible that an area of invasive carcinoma or other advanced histology was not removed. Hence, the presence of HGD in a conventional adenoma is worth reporting because it should lead to repeat endoscopy at a short interval to remove any residual lesion if there is any question about the completeness of excision of the initial lesion.

The third, and most reproducible, criterion for advanced adenoma is size. Size should be determined by the measurement at endoscopy rather than from a pathology report, given that adenomas are often taken out in a piecemeal fashion and that formalin fixation and handling may change the actual size of the lesion. Lesions 1 cm or greater in diameter are considered advanced adenomas. A majority of conventional adenomas with villous architecture are greater than 1 cm and in many studies size is a stronger predictor of recurrence than villous architecture.[15]

SERRATED POLYPS OF THE LARGE INTESTINE (HYPERPLASTIC POLYPS AND SERRATED ADENOMAS)

The most recent area of change in the classification of polyps of the large intestine has been in the area of serrated lesions, all of which were classified simply as HP before 1996.[16] Starting in 1996, new observations suggested that some lesions diagnosed as HPs had a propensity to develop into carcinoma, and one subtype, the SSA, is now recognized as the precursor lesion up to 35% of all colorectal carcinomas.[2,17] Given this fact, it is important for pathologists to be able to recognize these lesions and for clinicians to be aware of their occurrence and endoscopic appearance. Although the distinction of HP from SSA is now generally accepted, not all pathologists are familiar or comfortable with this diagnosis. Furthermore, there is considerable controversy over terminology, which has led to confusion for clinicians trying to understand these lesions and make sense of the literature, and there are still issues in regard to reproducibility of diagnosis and natural history that remain to be resolved.

HPs, which account for about 80% of all serrated lesions, are small, pearly white sessile lesions typically located in the sigmoid colon and rectum although they may occur anywhere in the colon. HPs are often present in clusters, and may safely be left in place although biopsy sampling of a few lesions to confirm the diagnosis of HP is often done. Microscopically they have straight crypts with retention of proliferation in the base of the crypts as occurs in normal mucosa (**Fig. 4**).[17,18] The subtypes of HPs (microvesicular and others) are theoretically important and may someday play a role in management, but at the current time do not have any particular therapeutic

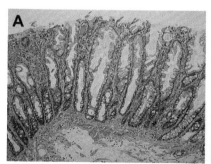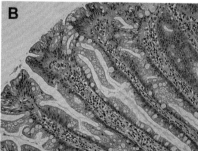

Fig. 4. HP (microvesicular type). (*A*) At low power, the lesion shows straight crypts with relatively narrow bases and with increasing serration as near the luminal surface (*top*). (*B*) The cells are not dysplastic and contain a mixture of goblet cells and microvesicular mucin.

implications and are not usually included in diagnosis. HPs do not have cytologic atypia (ie, dysplasia). The finding of typical HPs does not require a shortened surveillance interval.

SSAs (also reported in the literature as sessile serrated polyps and serrated polyps with abnormal architecture) appear as flat ill-defined lesions the color of the surrounding mucosa, often with adherent mucus or stool. Careful washing away of mucus or stool adherent to the mucosa, particularly in the right colon, may allow visualization of lesions that would otherwise be missed. SSAs account for 15% to 25% of all serrated lesions and in one large study were found in 9% of patients undergoing colonoscopy.[19] SSAs are more likely to be identified in the right colon, although even in the right colon the majority of serrated polyps, especially the smaller ones, are HPs. Therefore, it is more important to excise all lesions in the right colon than in the left. Microscopically, SSAs are characterized by abnormalities in proliferation with the proliferative zone no longer located at the base of the crypts. This abnormality leads to an architectural distortion with abnormally shaped crypts often showing excessive serration, sometimes referred to as architectural dysplasia (**Fig. 5**). SSAs are characterized by mutations of the BRAF gene, as are microvesicular HPs.[4] SSAs also demonstrate extensive methylation of the promoter region of several genes, including MLH1. SSAs do not have overt cytologic dysplasia of the type seen in conventional adenomas, which is the reason some investigators prefer the designation sessile serrated polyp for these lesions. Cytologic dysplasia does develop after methylation of the MLH1 gene, at which point these lesions are MSI and prone to rapid progression to carcinoma (**Fig. 6**).[20,21] The fact that these lesions are predominantly located in the right colon correlates with the preponderance of MSI carcinomas in that location, and the BRAF mutations in SSA explains why most sporadic MSI carcinomas (as opposed to MSI carcinomas as part of Lynch syndrome) are BRAF mutated. Lesions that are MSI and demonstrate cytologic dysplasia are referred to as SSA with cytologic dysplasia and not as mixed SSA–tubular adenomas because the mechanism of the dysplasia is totally different from that of conventional adenomas (which are usually mutated at the APC gene and are MSS). The term, *mixed SSA–tubular adenoma*, is not recommended because it fails to convey the potential for rapid progression to carcinoma, which can occur with an SSA with cytologic dysplasia (and the need for short-interval surveillance, discussed later).

The lesion referred to as TSA, also reported in the literature as filiform serrated adenoma and sometimes simply as serrated adenoma, is a rare lesion (constituting

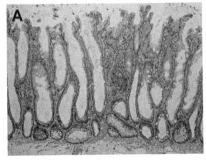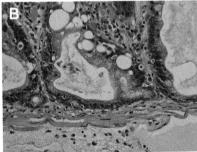

Fig. 5. SSA. (*A*) At low power, the crypts are distorted and the base of many of the crypts are dilated and L- or boot shaped. (*B*) Base of a crypt demonstrating dilation of the crypt and mature mucin-containing cells in a location where only proliferative cells are seen in a HP.

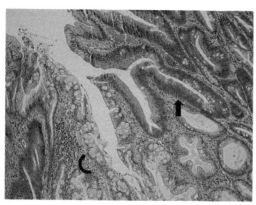

Fig. 6. SSA with dysplasia. This lesion shows features of SSA (*curved arrow*) adjacent to cytologically dysplastic areas resembling conventional adenoma (*straight arrow*).

<1% of colonic polyps) occurring as a large sessile polyp almost exclusively in the sigmoid colon or rectum. TSA is characterized by loss of polarity of the crypts with the formation of ectopic crypts and very elongated villiform structures.[16,18] There is a peculiar cell lining the surface of many of these lesions that is a senescent but cytologically abnormal cell (**Fig. 7**). These lesions are often misdiagnosed as conventional villous adenomas. TSA does become malignant but is not MSI; the type of carcinoma it leads to is currently unknown, although it may be a CIMP+ carcinoma with low levels of MSI due to methylation of the MGMT gene.[2] TSA is sometimes referred to only as serrated adenoma, a term that is ambiguous in that it has been used for TSA as well as for SSA with cytologic dysplasia, lesions that are different. Therefore, it is now recommended that serrated adenoma without a qualifier never be used.[16,18,22] If a gastroenterologist encounters such a diagnosis in a pathology report it is important to contact the pathologist to find out exactly what lesion the pathologist is referring to. Little is known about the natural history of TSA. There is no reason to believe that TSA is any more aggressive than conventional adenoma; at the current time my recommendations for TSA mirror those for conventional adenoma. Because most TSAs are

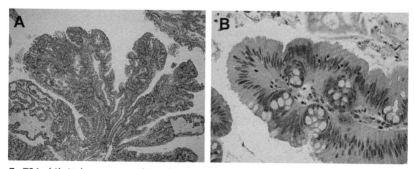

Fig. 7. TSA. (*A*) At low power, these lesions tend to be very exophytic with long fronds of tissue resembling villi. (*B*) The cell lining many of the fronds is a senescent cell with brightly eosinophilic cytoplasm. These cells do not resemble the dysplastic cells of conventional adenoma (**Fig. 1**). Also note the small abortive crypts emanating from the surface, a characteristic feature of TSA.

greater than 1 cm in size, follow-up screening as for other advanced adenomas is recommended.

Patients with multiple serrated lesions may have serrated polyposis, a form of polyposis previously known as hyperplasic polyposis. Hyperplastic polyposis is now recognized as a misnomer, because the majority of the polyps seen in these patients are SSAs rather than HPs.[22,23] The current definition for serrated polyposis is (1) at least five serrated polyps proximal to the sigmoid colon with two or more of them larger than 10 mm, (2) any number of serrated polyps proximal to the sigmoid colon in an individual who has a first-degree relative with serrated polyposis, or (3) more than 20 serrated polyps of any size, distributed throughout the colon.[22] Recently, multiple SSAs have also been reported in patients with MYH polyposis, although this remains to be confirmed.[24]

RECOMMENDED SURVEILLANCE INTERVALS FOR SESSILE SERRATED ADENOMAS

Given the relatively recent description of SSA and ongoing confusion about terminology, little is known about the recurrence rate or natural history of these lesions. There are no long-term follow-up studies for SSA as there are for conventional adenomas. Recently proposed clinical guidelines that include serrated adenomas do not clearly define what it meant by serrated adenoma, hence are of no real value. At the current time, recommendations are based on an understanding of the molecular mechanisms of carcinogenesis in these lesions combined with anecdotal clinical observations.[16,25] This information includes the following:

1. SSAs develop into carcinoma in a stepwise process that probably starts with a mutation of the BRAF gene and is followed by the accumulation of transcription errors caused by methylation of several genes. For the development of MSI carcinoma, when the MLH1 gene is methylated, the lesion converts to MSI status concurrently with the development of cytologic dysplasia. At this point the lesion is at high risk for the development of carcinoma. The mechanism by which SSA converts to CIMP+, MSS carcinoma is not known but presumably involves methylation of other critical genes and the rate of progression to malignancy is not known.
2. Most SSAs seem to grow to a large size without developing cytologic dysplasia; therefore, methylation of MLH1 seems uncommon.
3. In distinction from item 2, there are rare SSAs that develop into carcinoma while small (<1 cm), indicating that although methylation of MLH1 is an uncommon event, it probably is a random event and can occur at any stage in the development of the lesion.[20,21] These small polyps with early MLH1 methylation may account for interval cancers and lead to significant difficulties in predicting what might happen with an individual lesion.
4. SSAs may be difficult to visualize with routine colonoscopy and may be missed or incompletely removed. This failure to recognize/remove SSAs may account for the development of interval cancers from these lesions.[7,8]

Based on these factors, the following recommendations have been made[16,25]:

1. All SSAs should be completely removed if possible. For patients with a completely removed SSA without cytologic dysplasia, given the current uncertainty of the recurrence rate of these lesions and that they may be difficult to completely excise, repeat endoscopy at a short interval (3 years) should be considered.

2. For patients with SSA without cytologic dysplasia that are not completely removed, an attempt should be made for complete endoscopic excision. If this is not possible, repeat annual colonoscopy with extensive biopsy should be considered to evaluate possible evolution of the disease and development of cytologic dysplasia, at which point excision by any means is recommended if possible. For patients unwilling to undergo repeat endoscopy, surgical excision of the SSA without cytologic dysplasia may be appropriate, especially if the lesion is large or if a patient has multiple lesions (see serrated polyposis management, discussed later).

3. All SSAs with cytologic dysplasia should be completely removed. If a lesion cannot be removed endoscopically, then surgical excision should be considered. After endoscopic removal of SSA with cytologic dysplasia, repeat endoscopy at 1 year to evaluate possible recurrence of disease is recommended. This recommendation is based on the fact that SSAs are difficult to visualize and remove completely; hence, it seems important to assure that there is no regrowth of these high-risk lesions. If no lesion is identified at the 1-year repeat examination, then the patient can move to 1- or 3-year screening as for SSA without cytologic dysplasia depending on the number of SSAs detected (see item 7).

4. Patients with serrated (hyperplastic) polyposis present a unique challenge. The rate of development of carcinoma does not seem great enough to warrant prophylactic colectomy; however, the risk of malignancy is significant. Therefore, an attempt should be made to remove as many lesions as is reasonable, looking for cytologic dysplasia or carcinoma. If SSAs with cytologic dysplasia are identified, then consideration should be given to surgical excision of the colon. Because MSI carcinomas have a predilection for right-sided occurrence, it may be adequate to perform a subtotal colectomy with close follow-up of the small amount of residual colon rather than performing a total proctocolectomy.

5. For patients with multiple documented SSAs but not fulfilling the criteria for serrated polyposis, consideration should be given to annual screening to reduce the incidence of interval carcinomas.

INVASIVE CARCINOMA IN ADENOMA

When invasive carcinoma arises in an adenoma, additional management issues come into play.[26] Most of what is known about management of invasive carcinoma in adenoma is known only for carcinomas arising in conventional adenomas. Carcinoma in SSA is discussed later. Factors affecting management include the type of adenoma, particularly if it is pedunculated or sessile, the type of carcinoma, the presence of vascular invasion, and the status of the resection margin. Pedunculated lesions are more easily treated with local excision than sessile lesions, but it is not always possible for a pathologist to determine if a polyp was pedunculated or not unless there is a considerable stalk on the polyp. Endoscopic excision is considered adequate if (1) the invasive tumor is well or moderately differentiated (low-grade) adenocarcinoma, (2) there is no evidence of lymphatic or blood vessel invasion, and (3) the resection margin is negative for malignancy (which assumes that the specimen it oriented well enough to evaluate the margin). If any of these factors is not present, then further excision is recommended. Factors that may play a role in the extent of further excision include the location of the polyp, the general health and life expectancy of the patient, and the depth of invasion in the portion of carcinoma resected.

Management of carcinoma arising in SSA is less well characterized than for conventional adenoma; however, in my experience, carcinomas arising in SSA are not generally amenable to endoscopic resection. The main reason for this may be as simple as the shape of the SSA. SSAs are flat lesions and are not particularly amenable to total endoscopic resection as a single polyp. When carcinoma arises in an SSA it almost immediately grows into the submucosa and is often considerably deeper, perhaps because these lesions tend to be detected late or perhaps because of the rapid progression to carcinoma once the lesion becomes MSI. Most carcinomas arising in SSAs in my experience have been taken out piecemeal; further therapy is essentially always required.

LYNCH SYNDROME AND MSI TESTING

There has been much interest in recent years regarding testing for MSI in colorectal adenocarcinoma. This is mainly because of the occurrence of MSI in tumors associated with Lynch syndrome. Identification of patients with Lynch syndrome is important not only for the patient (because knowing that a patient has Lynch syndrome changes the surgical approach to the colon resection and puts the patient at high risk of other Lynch-associated malignancies) but also for the patient's family, who require more intense screening if identified as having the mutation for Lynch syndrome. Identification of MSI is also important for prognosis, because MSI carcinoma (sporadic as well as Lynch associated) has a better prognosis than MSS carcinoma and may be important for selecting chemotherapeutic agents.

Testing for MSI can be done with two methods, immunohistochemistry (IHC), looking for the MMR gene products, or polymerase chain reaction (PCR)-based testing directly for MSI (ie, variation in the length of microsatellite segments).[27] Details of the testing methods are beyond the scope of this article. Briefly, however, IHC testing involves staining of paraffin-embedded tissue looking directly for loss of MMR genes, whereas PCR testing for MSI involves removing tissue from paraffin blocks and comparing the size of specific microsatellite segments from the tumor with those from nontumorous tissue from the same patient. The advantages of IHC testing are that it is generally available in any large pathology laboratory, it identifies the gene likely responsible for the MSI, and it can be done on a biopsy and does not require normal tissue for comparison. Disadvantages include a false-negative rate in the range of 2%, which can be either technical or because of mutations that allow for a nonfunctional but antigenically intact gene product, and that it might be considered a genetic test requiring patient permission to perform.[28] Advantages of PCR-based MSI testing include high sensitivity (although there is a false-negative rate of approximately 2% with PCR as well, usually on the basis of sampling error) and the fact that this is usually not considered a genetic test and can be performed without patient permission. Disadvantages include requiring a dedicated molecular diagnostics laboratory and normal tissue from the patient needed for comparison with the tumor tissue, which means that this test cannot be performed on small biopsies or polyps. In addition, a positive result for MSI by PCR does not allow determination of which gene is involved and is almost always followed up by IHC testing, increasing the overall cost of testing. The most effective testing scheme is to do IHC first, and if all MMR genes are intact do PCR-based MSI testing only if the index of suspicion for Lynch syndrome is high.[28] MSI testing by either method does not absolutely differentiate sporadic MSI tumors from Lynch syndrome, particularly if the missing gene product is MLH1 (absence of MSH2, MSH6, or PMS2 products usually does imply Lynch syndrome). For patients missing their MLH1 gene, testing for BRAF mutation is helpful, because mutation of BRAF indicates a sporadic lesion rather than Lynch syndrome.[2]

For a gastroenterologist, the issue of MSI testing of biopsies or polypectomy specimens showing carcinoma before surgery is an important consideration. If patients have Lynch syndrome, they are likely to benefit from a more extensive colonic resection for the carcinoma than is necessary for patients with a sporadic non–Lynch syndrome carcinoma. Therefore, testing of the malignant biopsy/polypectomy by IHC can be useful in determining the appropriate surgical approach to a patient.

One question that often comes up in patients with a family history of colon carcinoma is whether or not testing of a conventional adenoma without carcinoma can be used to diagnose Lynch syndrome. Adenomas in patients with Lynch syndrome may be either MSS or MSI, depending on the status of the second MMR allele in the patient. If a second hit has occurred in the adenoma, then the adenoma demonstrates loss of MMR and is diagnostic of Lynch syndrome. Alternatively, not all adenomas in Lynch syndrome patients demonstrate loss of MMR; the presence of intact MMRs in an adenoma does not mean that a patient does not have Lynch syndrome. Therefore, testing of adenomas may be useful in confirming a diagnosis of Lynch syndrome but cannot be used to rule out the diagnosis and is of limited usefulness.

Other questions with MSI testing are, Who should be tested? and Which permissions are necessary before testing? Both of these are controversial topics. The most recognized criteria for testing are the Bethesda guidelines.[29] Recent data, however, indicate that using the Bethesda guidelines miss as many as 20% of all Lynch syndrome patients, leading to the alternative suggestion of testing all newly diagnosed colon carcinoma cases for MSI, with appropriate secondary work-up if the case turns out to be MSI.[28,29] Some institutions have opted to test all new carcinomas without specific patient permission, rationalizing that this is just part of patient care similar to examining a liver biopsy for α_1-antitrypsin deficiency, whereas others have argued that testing using IHC for MMR proteins cannot be performed without patient permission. MSI testing by PCR, alternatively, does not look at specific gene products and the majority of cases detected to be MSI positive are sporadic, not constituting a genetic test. At this time there seems to be no consensus about routine testing versus testing only with specific consent; the final decision will be up to local legal guidelines.

REFERENCES

1. Fearon ER, Vogelstein B. A genetic model for colorectal tumorigenesis. Cell 1990; 61:759–67.
2. Jass JR. Classification of colorectal cancer based on correlation of clinical, morphological and molecular features. Histopathology 2007;50:113–30.
3. Jass JR, Whitehall VL, Young J, et al. Emerging concepts in colorectal neoplasia. Gastroenterology 2002;123:862–76.
4. O'Brien MJ, Yang S, Mack C, et al. Comparison of microsatellite instability, CpG island methylation phenotype, BRAF and KRAS status in serrated polyps and traditional adenomas indicates separate pathways to distinct colorectal carcinoma end points. Am J Surg Pathol 2006;30:1491–501.
5. Rabeneck L, Davila JA, El-Serag HB. Is there a true "shift" to the right colon in the incidence of colorectal cancer? Am J Gastroenterol 2003;98:1400–9.
6. Brenner H, Hoffmeister M, Arndt V, et al. Protection from right- and left-sided colorectal neoplasms after colonoscopy: population-based study. J Natl Cancer Inst 2010;102:89–95.

7. Sawhney MS, Farrar WD, Gudiseva S, et al. Microsatellite instability in interval colon cancers. Gastroenterology 2006;131:1700–5.
8. Arain MA, Sawhney M, Sheikh S, et al. CIMP status of interval colon cancers: another piece to the puzzle. Am J Gastroenterol 2010;105(5):1189–95.
9. Winawer SJ, Zauber AG, Fletcher RH, et al. Guidelines for colonoscopy surveillance after polypectomy: a consensus update by the US Multi-Society Task Force on Colorectal Cancer and the American Cancer Society. CA Cancer J Clin 2006;56:143–59.
10. Rex DK, Johnson DA, Anderson JC, et al. American College of Gastroenterology guidelines for colorectal cancer screening 2008. Am J Gastroenterol 2009;104: 739–50.
11. Laiyemo AO, Murphy G, Albert PS, et al. Postpolypectomy surveillance guidelines: predictive accuracy for advanced adenoma at 4 years. Ann Intern Med 2008;148:419–26.
12. Appelman HD. CON: high-grade dysplasia and villous features should not be part of the routine diagnosis of colorectal adenomas. Am J Gastroenterol 2008; 103:1329–31.
13. Rex DK, Goldblum JR. PRO: villous elements and high-grade dysplasia help guide post-polypectomy colonoscopic surveillance. Am J Gastroenterol 2008; 103:1327–9.
14. Lindgren G, Liljegren A, Jaramillo E, et al. Adenoma prevalence and cancer risk in familial non-polyposis colorectal cancer. Gut 2002;50:228–34.
15. Martinez ME, Baron JA, Lieberman DA, et al. A pooled analysis of advanced colorectal neoplasia diagnoses after colonoscopic polypectomy. Gastroenterology 2009;136:832–41.
16. Snover DC. Serrated polyps of the large intestine. Semin Diagn Pathol 2005;22: 301–8.
17. Torlakovic E, Skovland E, Snover DC, et al. Morphologic reappraisal of serrated colorectal polyps. Am J Surg Pathol 2003;27:65–81.
18. Torlakovic EE, Gomez JD, Driman DK, et al. Sessile serrated adenoma (SSA) vs. traditional serrated adenoma (TSA). Am J Surg Pathol 2008;32:21–9.
19. Spring KJ, Zhao ZZ, Walsh MD, et al. High prevalence of sessile serrated adenomas with BRAF mutations: a prospective study of patients undergoing colonoscopy. Gastroenterology 2006;131:1400–7.
20. Goldstein NS. Small colonic microsatellite unstable carcinomas and high grade epithelial dysplasias in sessile serrated adenoma polypectomy specimens. A study of eight cases. Am J Clin Pathol 2006;125:132–45.
21. Sheridan TB, Fenton H, Lewin MR, et al. Sessile serrated adenomas with low- and high-grade dysplasia and early carcinomas: an immunohistochemical study of serrated lesions "caught in the act". Am J Clin Pathol 2006;126:564–71.
22. Snover DC, Ahnen DJ, Burt RW, et al. Serrated polyps of the colon and rectum and serrated ("hyperplastic") polyposis. In: Bozman FT, Carneiro F, Hruban RH, et al, editors. WHO classification of tumours. Pathology and genetics. Tumours of the digestive system. 4th edition. Berlin: Springer-Verlag; 2010.
23. Torlakovic E, Snover DC. Serrated adenomatous polyposis in humans. Gastroenterology 1996;110:748–55.
24. Boparai KS, Dekker E, Van Eeden S, et al. Hyperplastic polyps and sessile serrated adenomas as a phenotypic expression of MYH-associated polyposis. Gastroenterology 2008;135:2014–8.
25. East JE, Saunders BP, Jass JR. Sporadic and syndromic hyperplastic polyps and serrated adenomas of the colon:classification, molecular genetics, natural history, and clinical management. Gastroenterol Clin North Am 2008;37:25–46.

26. Bond JH. Polyp guideline: diagnosis, treatment, and surveillance for patients with colorectal polyps. Am J Gastroenterol 2000;95:3053–63.

27. Burgart LJ. Testing for defective DNA mismatch repair in colorectal carcinoma: a practical guide. Arch Pathol Lab Med 2005;129:1385–9.

28. Hampel H, Frankel WL, Martin E, et al. Screening for the Lynch syndrome (hereditary nonpolyposis colorectal cancer). N Engl J Med 2005;352:1851–60.

29. Julié C, Trésallet C, Brouquet A, et al. Identification in daily practice of patients with lynch syndrome (hereditary nonpolyposis colorectal cancer): revised Bethesda guidelines-based approach *versus* molecular screening. Am J Gastroenterol 2008;103:2825–35.

Complications of Colonoscopy: Magnitude and Management

Cynthia W. Ko, MD, MS[a], Jason A. Dominitz, MD, MHS[b],*

KEYWORDS

- Colonoscopy complications • Quality improvement program
- Gastrointestinal bleeding • Colonic perforation

Although complications of colonoscopy are rare, they are potentially quite serious and life threatening. In addition, less serious adverse events may occur frequently and may have an impact on a patient's willingness to undergo future procedures, as might be required in a colonoscopic surveillance program. This article reviews the magnitude of and risk factors for major and minor colonoscopy complications, discusses management of complications, and suggests ways to design quality improvement programs to reduce the risk of complications. Studies of colonoscopic complications are generally limited by retrospective data collection methods and under-reporting of complications. This is particularly true of less serious adverse events and single-institution studies (where patients experiencing complications may seek medical attention at another facility). Furthermore, there are variable definitions of adverse events, making comparison of complications rates across studies problematic.

SERIOUS GASTROINTESTINAL COLONOSCOPY COMPLICATIONS

Many studies have reported the risks of serious colonoscopy complications, and most commonly have tracked the risks of colonic perforation or gastrointestinal bleeding.[1–28] Other serious complications include postpolypectomy syndrome and

Funding Source: American Society for Gastrointestinal Endoscopy Endoscopic Research Career Development Award (JAD). This material is based on work supported by the VA Puget Sound Health Care System, Department of Veterans Affairs. The views expressed in this article are those of the authors and do not necessarily reflect the position or policy of the Department of Veterans Affairs.

[a] Department of Medicine, Division of Gastroenterology, University of Washington, Box 356424, Seattle, WA, USA

[b] VA Puget Sound Health Care System, Department of Medicine, Division of Gastroenterology, University of Washington, 1660 South Columbian Way (111-S-Gastro), Seattle, WA 98108, USA

* Corresponding author.

E-mail address: Jason.dominitz@va.gov

diverticulitis. It is known that serious complications, in particular gastrointestinal bleeding, can occur at delayed intervals (up to 3–4 weeks postcolonoscopy), and complication rates need to be tracked at least until this time point.

A summary of the findings of prior large studies of colonoscopy complications is shown in **Table 1**. In general, the risk of colonic perforation has been most thoroughly studied. Although this is potentially the most serious complication, it is also uncommon, with reported rates from large studies of less than 0.3% and generally less than 0.1%. Lower gastrointestinal bleeding is the most common serious complication, with reported risk between 0.1% and 0.6%. Postpolypectomy syndrome, where use of electrocautery results in a transmural burn and localized peritonitis, is infrequently studied but also seems uncommon (<0.2%). Diverticulitis has also been reported as a serious complication of colonoscopy, with an incidence ranging from 0.04% to 0.08%. The reported risk of death after colonoscopy varies between 0 and 0.09%.

It is unclear whether or not the risk of complications is less with colonoscopy for screening or surveillance indications than with colonoscopy for diagnostic indications. In a systematic review, the US Preventive Services Task Force estimated the incidence of serious complications after screening colonoscopy in predominantly asymptomatic persons to be 2.8 per 1000 examinations (95% CI, 1.5–5.2).[29] In a study of Medicare beneficiaries, Warren and colleagues[14] found a lower risk of serious gastrointestinal complications after screening colonoscopy (2.4/1000 examinations) than after diagnostic colonoscopy (4.2/1000 examinations) or after colonoscopy with polypectomy (9.3/1000 examinations).

LESS SEVERE ADVERSE EVENTS

Because most previous studies have focused on major complications after colonoscopy, the risks of less serious complications, such as self-limited bleeding or abdominal pain, are even less clearly documented.[11,16,30] A substantial proportion of patients (up 33%), however, report some gastrointestinal symptoms after colonoscopy.[11,16,30] Reported symptoms include abdominal pain (10.5%), bloating (25%), self-limited gastrointestinal bleeding (3.8%), diarrhea (6.3%), and nausea (4.0%). These symptoms generally are mild and resolve within 2 days after colonoscopy.

SEDATION-RELATED AND CARDIOVASCULAR COMPLICATIONS

Serious complications from moderate sedation for colonoscopy are also uncommon but include respiratory depression, hypoxia, chest pain, cardiac arrhythmias, hypo- or hypertension, and vasovagal reactions. McQuaid and Laine,[31] in a meta-analysis of randomized trials for moderate sedation, found a risk of hypoxemia of 18% for patients receiving midazolam alone versus 11% for patients receiving midazolam with a narcotic. In analysis of data from 174,255 colonoscopies in the Clinical Outcomes Research Initiative (CORI) database, Sharma and colleagues[32] found an overall risk of cardiopulmonary complications after colonoscopy of 1100/100,000 procedures. The most common cardiopulmonary complications were transient hypoxia (230/100,000 procedures), bradycardia (280/100,000 procedures), hypotension (480/100,000 procedures), and vasovagal reactions (190/100,000 procedures). Oxygen supplementation was required in 7650/100,000 procedures) and intravenous fluids in 310/100,000 procedures. Reversal of sedation occurred in 490/100,000 procedures. Higher American Society of Anesthesiologists class and increasing age were significant independent predictors of cardiovascular events related to sedation, and adverse events were more common for inpatient than for outpatient procedures. The dose of midazolam used was inversely associated with risk for cardiovascular events.

Table 1
Summary of studies of colonoscopy complications

	Study Setting	Number of Examinations	Death	Perforation	Gastrointestinal Bleeding N (%)	Postpolypectomy Syndrome
Levin et al, 2006[12]	Diagnostic and screening colonoscopy in Kaiser Permanente system	16,318	10 (0.06%)	15 (0.09%)	53 (0.32%)	6 (0.04%)
Warren et al, 2009[14]	Medicare claims data	53,220	53 (0.09%)	33 (0.06%)	340 (0.64%)	NR
Ko et al, 2009[10]	Screening and surveillance colonoscopy in CORI network	21,375	2 (0.01%)	4 (0.02%)	34 (0.16%)	2 (0.01%)
Rabeneck et al, 2008[13]	Canadian claims data	97,091	5 (0.07%)	58 (0.08%)	137 (0.16%)	NR
Imperiale et al, 2000[6]	Screening colonoscopy study	2686	0 (0%)	1 (0.04%)	3 (0.1%)	NR
Mandel et al, 1993[15]	Colonoscopy for follow-up of positive fecal occult blood test	12,246	NR	4 (0.03%)	11 (0.1%)	NR
Viiala et al, 2003[1]	Australian teaching hospital	23,508	3 (0.01%)	23 (0.1%)	49 (0.2%)	22 (0.1%)
Gatto et al, 2003[9]	SEER-Medicare data	39,286	4 (0.01%)	77 (0.2%)	NR	NR
Korman et al, 2003[9]	Network of US ambulatory surgery centers	116,000	NR	37 (0.3%)	NR	NR
Anderson et al, 2000[3]	US teaching hospital	10,486	2 (0.02%)	20 (0.2%)	NR	NR
Nelson et al, 2002[4]	VA cooperative study, screening colonoscopy	3196	0 (0%)	0 (0%)	6 (0.2%)	NR
Sieg et al, 2001[4]	Germany	82,416	2 (0.001%)	13 (0.01%)	38 (0.05%)	5 (0.003%)
Tran et al, 2001[18]	US teaching hospital	26,162	1 (0.004%)	21 (0.08%)	NR	NR
Rathgaber and Wick, 2006[25]	US community practice	12,407	0 (0%)	2 (0.01%)	25 (0.22%)	NR
Johnson et al, 2008[24]	CT colonography study	2531	NR	NR	1 (0.03%)	NR
Farley et al, 1997[26]	Mayo Clinic	57,028	NR	43 (0.08%)	NR	NR
Luning et al, 2007[28]	Dutch teaching hospital	30,366	NR	35 (0.12%)	NR	NR
Iqbal et al, 2005[27]	Mayo Clinic	78,702	72 (0.08%)	NR	NR	NR

Complications were variably defined across studies and length of follow-up differed.
Abbreviations: NR, not reported; SEER, Surveillance, Epidemiology and End Results Program.

Additional concerns have arisen over the potential risk of excess cardiovascular events within 30 days of colonoscopy. Warren and colleagues[14] examined the risk of cardiovascular events in Medicare beneficiaries after colonoscopy and found a modestly increased risk of cardiovascular events requiring an emergency visit or hospitalization after colonoscopy compared with a cohort matched on age, gender, and comorbidity (unadjusted overall risk 19.4/1000 vs 16.6/1000, P<.001). The most common adverse cardiovascular event was arrhythmia (10.2/1000). This increased risk of cardiovascular events seemed most pronounced for patients who had a polypectomy (adjusted risk 23.3/1000 persons) compared with matched patients who did not undergo colonoscopy (adjusted risk 15.9/1000) or patients who underwent screening colonoscopy (adjusted risk 12.5/1000) or diagnostic colonoscopy (adjusted risk 15.8/1000). The presence of comorbidities, including diabetes, stroke, atrial fibrillation, or congestive heart failure, was associated with increased risk of cardiovascular events compared with patients without these comorbidities. The risk of cardiovascular events, however, was not significantly different from matched control groups who did not undergo colonoscopy. Another study of screening and surveillance colonoscopy, with generally younger patients, did not find an excess risk of cardiovascular events.[10]

COMPLICATIONS RELATED TO BOWEL PREPARATION

Bowel preparation regimens fall into two general categories: electrolyte solutions containing polyethylene glycol (PEG) (eg, GoLYTELY, Colyte, and NuLYTELY) and non-PEG solutions, including sodium phosphate solutions (eg, Fleet's Phospho-Soda, OsmoPrep, and Visicol). Although lower-volume sodium phosphate preparations are often better tolerated, concerns have arisen about renal injury after these preparations.[33,34] These preparations are hyperosmotic and can lead to fluid retention, leading to concerns about their use in patients with underlying cardiac, renal, or hepatic diseases. Studies of healthy adults undergoing colonoscopy have shown development of significant hypocalcemia or hyperphosphatemia.[35] Most concerning is the risk of developing acute phosphate nephropathy due to precipitation of calcium-phosphate crystals in the kidney. The risk of acute phosphate nephropathy may be increased in the elderly or in those who are inadequately hydrated. Risk may also increase with hypertension or with use of certain antihypertensive medications, including diuretics, angiotensin-converting enzyme (ACE) inhibitors, or angiotensin receptor blockers (ARBs).[34]

The overall risk of acute phosphate nephropathy is unknown but is estimated at less than 0.1%.[34] In a retrospective study, Hurst and colleagues[36] found acute kidney injury, defined as an increase in serum creatinine of greater than 0.5 mg/dL, in 1.2% of patients within 12 months of colonoscopy. Acute kidney injury was more common in patients who had received a sodium phosphate preparation compared with PEG-based solutions (1.3% vs 0.9%, P<0.001). Additional risk factors for acute kidney injury in this study included older age and congestive heart failure. Brunelli and colleagues[37] found a risk of acute kidney injury only in patients who are also receiving ACE inhibitors or ARBs. Despite these concerns about sodium phosphate preparations, other retrospective studies have found similar proportions of patients who develop renal insufficiency after colonoscopy with sodium phosphate or PEG-based preparations.[38,39]

Because of these reports, oral sodium phosphate solutions have fallen out of favor for bowel preparation, and the Food and Drug Administration has issued a safety warning about these drugs.[40] Use of sodium phosphate preparations is not advised in elderly patients, those with pre-existing kidney disease, and those with pre-existing fluid or electrolyte imbalances, such as patients with congestive heart failure. The importance of adequate hydration with these preparations has also been emphasized.

PEG-based solutions do not lead to substantial shifts in fluid levels and can be safely used for patients with electrolyte imbalances, congestive heart failure, or chronic kidney disease.[41] Because of the large volume of the preparation required, however, they are often difficult for patients to tolerate. Symptoms of nausea/vomiting and abdominal fullness are common during ingestion. Less common complications associated with large-volume preparations include vomiting-induced Mallory-Weiss tears,[42] esophageal rupture,[43] pulmonary aspiration,[44] hypothermia, and cardiac arrhythmias.[45,46] Although reported, electrolyte abnormalities are less common with PEG-based solutions than with sodium phosphate preparations.[47]

MISCELLANEOUS COMPLICATIONS

Miscellaneous and rare complications of colonoscopy include splenic hematoma or rupture,[48] acute appendicitis,[49] incarcerated hernias,[50] subcutaneous emphysema in the absence of perforation,[51] intramural hematoma,[52] and ischemic colitis.[53] Colonic explosions have been reported with electrocautery in patients with suboptimal bowel preparation,[54] in particular with mannitol preparations, which are not currently used. Although transient bacteremia occurs frequently after colonoscopy,[55] complications of bacteremia, such as infective endocarditis, are rare, and antibiotic prophylaxis is not routinely recommended.[56,57] If glutaraldehyde is used in the endoscope disinfection process, a chemical colitis can occur if the endoscope has not been adequately rinsed before the next procedure.[58]

RISK FACTORS FOR SERIOUS COLONOSCOPY COMPLICATIONS

Increasing age has consistently been found a significant risk factor for serious gastrointestinal events after colonoscopy.[8,12–14] For example, Gatto and colleagues[8] found a nearly 4-fold increased risk of perforation for subjects aged 75 to 79 years compared with those aged 65 to 69 years (odds ratio [OR] 3.5; 95% CI, 1.5–7.8). Female gender may be a risk factor for colonic perforation in particular.[9,12] This may related to the finding that colonoscopy is generally more difficult in women than in men, likely due to pelvic anatomy and prior pelvic surgery, which is more common in women.[59,60] Although the presence of comorbid conditions, such as diabetes, stroke, atrial fibrillation, and congestive heart failure, has been associated with increased risk of serious adverse events in the Medicare population,[8,14] this association has not been found consistently in all studies.[10,13]

The risk of complications increases markedly in examinations where a polypectomy is performed, in particular with use of electrocautery.[10,12–14] Levin and colleagues[12] found a 9-fold increased risk of any serious complication in colonoscopies where a biopsy or polypectomy was performed (OR 9.2; 95% CI, 2.9–29.0), although the risk of perforation alone was not significantly increased (OR 1.9; 95% CI, 0.3–10.9). The risk of complications, most commonly gastrointestinal bleeding, increases further if more than one polypectomy with electrocautery is performed[10] and with larger polyp size.[12] Biopsy alone may also increase the risk of complications.[12] Prior studies have suggested that hot biopsy for removal of polyps is associated with increased bleeding risk, particularly if used in the proximal colon.[61–63]

Although some investigators hypothesize that endoscopist experience and skill may influence complication rates, there are few data to support or refute this possibility. In Canada, endoscopist specialty did not influence the risk of complications, but endoscopists with low colonoscopy volumes had higher risks of complications than high volume providers (OR 2.96 comparing lowest to highest quintile; 95% CI, 1.57–5.61).[13] When only including colonoscopies performed by gastroenterologists, however, colonoscopy volume was not associated with risk of complications. Studies are needed in other settings and countries to confirm these findings.

The use of warfarin or clopidogrel may also increase risk of colonoscopy complications,[64–66] in particular postpolypectomy bleeding. For example, Hui and colleagues[64] found that warfarin increased the risk of postpolypectomy bleeding (OR 13.37; 95% CI, 4.10–43.65), even after adjusting for other potential risk factors, such as patient age, location and size of polyp, polypectomy technique, and presence of underlying renal impairment. In contrast, use of aspirin or nonsteroidal anti-inflammatory medications has not been shown to increase the risk of postpolypectomy bleeding.[65–67] There are few published data about the risk of bleeding complications after use of clopidogrel.

Published guidelines recommend that management of anticoagulants and antiplatelet agents be individualized according to procedure risk and risks associated with the underlying condition.[68–70] For example, patients on warfarin therapy with low-risk conditions (such as nonvalvular atrial fibrillation, bioprosthetic valves, and mechanical valves in the aortic position) undergoing high-risk procedures (such as colonoscopy with polypectomy) should discontinue warfarin 3 to 5 days before the procedure. In patients with high-risk conditions (such as mechanical valves in the mitral position or valvular atrial fibrillation) undergoing high-risk procedures, warfarin should be discontinued 3 to 5 days before the procedure with consideration of bridging therapy with low molecular weight heparins. The effect of the timing of reinstitution of warfarin therapy on complication risk is also not well studied, but resumption of anticoagulation within 1 week of polypectomy seems to increase the risk of gastrointestinal bleeding (OR 5.2; 95% CI, 2.2–12.5).[66] Current guidelines recommend reinstituting therapy on the same night as the procedure, however, although delays can be considered if the polyps removed are large or otherwise at high risk for bleeding.

American Society of Gastrointestinal Endoscopy guidelines also suggest that aspirin or nonsteroidal anti-inflammatory drugs do not need to be discontinued for patients undergoing endoscopic procedures. Decisions about discontinuation of clopidogrel also need to be individualized according to the underlying indications for its use and the risks of the planned procedure.

PREVENTION OF COMPLICATIONS

It is an unfortunate truism that complications are inherent to the practice of endoscopy. Although colonoscopy offers a wide variety of diagnostic and therapeutic capabilities, careful selection of patients for colonoscopy can help minimize complications. For example, in patients at high risk for complications, less-invasive colonic imaging modalities (eg, CT colonography or barium enema) may be appropriate depending on the indication. When colonoscopy is indicated, there are techniques that have been suggested to reduce the complications. Given the overall low incidence of complications, however, high-quality studies proving the effectiveness of these techniques are generally absent. Therefore, most of these recommendations are based on expert opinion or low-quality studies.

Perforation in the setting of diagnostic colonoscopy may result from barotrauma (typically in the setting of a colonic stricture) or from mechanical trauma (as a result of loop formation with stretching of the colonic wall or by direct perforation by the colonoscope tip). The risk of barotrauma may be reduced by the judicious use of air during insufflation (or by substituting carbon dioxide insufflation).[71,72] Adherence to good insertion technique to minimize loop formation may help reduce mechanical perforation.[73]

As discussed previously, the risk of complications is significantly increased in patients undergoing therapeutic colonoscopy, typically polypectomy. Much has been written about proper polypectomy technique as endoscopists have endeavored to find means to prevent complications.[74,75] Because polypectomy-related perforation usually results from thermal injury to the colonic wall, use of cold techniques (eg, cold biopsy or snare resection without cautery) has been advocated for small nonpedunculated polyps.[74] For larger or pedunculated polyps, electrocautery is typically used to prevent bleeding. The use of pure low-power coagulation current presents a theoretically increased risk of perforation compared with blended or pure cut current, although there are no clinical data to support this contention.[74] Injection of saline or other agents into the submucosa has been used to lift sessile polyps and increase the separation of the colonic layers. Although this may reduce the risk of perforation, data to support this contention are limited.[76,77] Submucosal epinephrine injection may reduce the risk of postpolypectomy bleeding, especially for large or sessile polyps.[76,78] Some experts advocate pretreatment of pedunculated polyps with thick stalks with injection of epinephrine into the stalk, placement of a detachable snare on the stalk, or both.[78–80]

MANAGEMENT OF COMPLICATIONS
Patient Management

A detailed discussion of the management of colonoscopic complications is beyond the scope of this article, although general principles are addressed. All patients who experience a complication should be promptly managed by experienced medical personnel, often including a multidisciplinary team of endoscopists, interventional radiologists, and surgeons. Some complications are recognized at the time of endoscopy, and many can be endoscopically managed. For example, many cases of postpolypectomy bleeding can be controlled with mechanical hemostasis (eg, clips or detachable loops) or electrocautery techniques.[79,81] Small perforations noted at the time of endoscopy can sometimes be successfully closed with clips,[82,83] although careful observation is warranted and antibiotics may be appropriate. Generally, surgical consultation is also advised. For those complications that are not amenable to immediate endoscopic management, patients should be promptly admitted to a facility that is equipped to treat the complication, which may require medical, surgical, radiologic, or other interventions. Criteria for endoscopic, conservative, and surgical management of perforations have been proposed.[75]

Although most complications may be unavoidable, some do result from medical errors. Recently, increased attention has been focused on the disclosure of information to patients about medical errors, which has been defined by the Institute of Medicine as "failure of a planned action to be completed as intended, or the use of a wrong plan to achieve an aim."[84] Studies have shown that there is a gap between the expectation of patients for disclosure and apology and physicians' ability to effectively disclose errors.[85] Many institutions are adopting a policy of mandatory disclosure of medical errors, and since 2001, the Joint Commission requires disclosure of "unanticipated outcomes" as part of the accreditation standards for hospitals and health care organizations.[86] Although some clinicians may be concerned that disclosure will prompt patients to seek compensation through litigation, some evidence suggests that disclosure policies have resulted in fewer lawsuits.[85,87]

Practice Improvement

As part of an ongoing quality improvement program, individual physicians and groups should monitor complications on a regular basis. Endoscopists may not be aware of delayed colonoscopy complications unless specific efforts are made to determine if complications have occurred. Therefore, quality improvement programs should attempt to make specific efforts to identify adverse events for up to 30 days after colonoscopy. All complications should be reviewed and discussed with other providers in a structured quality improvement forum, such as a morbidity and mortality conference.[88] This forum should allow physicians to freely discuss the procedure and identify any processes of care that could have been improved. These conferences can also identify systematic issues that can be improved to impact quality of care. As part of a formal quality improvement process, these discussions are protected from medicolegal discovery. Benefits of this process include both the ability to identify systematic problems more quickly (eg, problems related to equipment malfunction or medication issues) as well as opportunities to improve patient care through sharing of expertise among providers.

Given the relatively rare occurrence of complications, it is typically necessary to review many months of procedures to reliably determine an individual endoscopist's complication rate. The incidence of complications should be measured for each procedure type (ie, all indications vs screening). Concern for inappropriate endoscopic practice is warranted for perforation rates that exceed 1 case in 500 overall colonoscopies or greater than 1 perforation in 1000 screening examinations.[89] Similarly, colonoscopic bleeding rates that exceed 1% should also be investigated.

The risk of complications is influenced by the patient population and the nature of the type of procedure that is performed. In some cases, there are concerns about the competence of a physician to perform colonoscopy as evidenced by an excessive complication rate. When minimal competence for the performance of colonoscopy is not assured, several options exist, including proctoring, continuing medical education, retraining, or limitation of privileges.[90]

Role of Specialty Societies in Reducing Complications

Given the infrequent nature of complications and the variability in patient populations, it is difficult for any individual or small group of endoscopists to identify risk factors for complications. Therefore, although individual endoscopists are responsible for the care they deliver to their patients, the community of endoscopists shares responsibility for helping determine the standards of practice for all patients to maximize the benefits of colonoscopy while minimizing harm. For example, the issue of management of antithrombotic therapy (eg, aspirin, clopidogrel, and warfarin) in the pericolonoscopy period is a controversial and evolving field. Gastroenterology specialty societies have modified their recommendations as new evidence becomes available concerning the risks of bleeding complications with continued antithrombotic therapy versus the risk of thromboembolic events with cessation of these medications.[68,69] Also, there has been considerable recent attention paid to potential infectious complications related to improper reprocessing of reusable medical equipment.[91] Gastroenterology specialty societies have taken an active role in educating their membership about identified problems and their corrective action as well as developing and updating guidelines for the reprocessing of endoscopes and accessories.[92,93] Specialty societies should continue to advocate for high standards for training of endoscopists and for ongoing research into methods to prevent colonoscopy complications.

SUMMARY

Complications are an unavoidable consequence of the practice of colonoscopy. Fortunately, these adverse events are relatively rare and their risk is generally outweighed by the beneficial diagnostic and therapeutic capabilities of colonoscopy for the vast majority of patients. Knowledge of potential complications, their risk factors, and the expected incidence can lead to improved risk-benefit analysis by physicians and patients and facilitate the performance of a comprehensive informed consent process. Early recognition of complications and prompt intervention is important to minimize patient morbidity. Quality improvement efforts help identify systematic problems that may be contributing to adverse events to improve patient outcomes.

REFERENCES

1. Viiala CH, Zimmerman M, Cullen DJ, et al. Complication rates of colonoscopy in an Australian teaching hospital environment. Intern Med J 2003;33(8):355–9.
2. Nivatvongs S. Complications in colonoscopic polypectomy: lessons to learn from an experience with 1576 polyps. Am Surg 1988;54(2):61–3.
3. Anderson ML, Pasha TM, Leighton JA. Endoscopic perforation of the colon: lessons from a 10-year study. Am J Gastroenterol 2000;95(12):3418–22.
4. Nelson DB, McQuaid KR, Bond JH, et al. Procedural success and complications of large-scale screening colonoscopy. Gastrointest Endosc 2002;55(3):307–14.
5. Sieg A, Hachmoeller-Eisenbach U, Eisenbach T. Prospective evaluation of complications in outpatient GI endoscopy: a survey among German gastroenterologists. Gastrointest Endosc 2001;53(6):620–7.
6. Imperiale TF, Wagner DR, Lin CY, et al. Risk of advanced proximal neoplasms in asymptomatic adults according to the distal colorectal findings. N Engl J Med 2000;343(3):169–74.
7. Levin TR, Zhao W, Conell C, et al. Complications of colonoscopy in a community practice setting. Gastroenterology 2004;126(Suppl 4):A25.
8. Gatto NM, Frucht H, Sundararajan V, et al. Risk of perforation after colonoscopy and sigmoidoscopy: a population-based study. J Natl Cancer Inst 2003;95(3): 230–6.
9. Korman LY, Overholt BF, Box T, et al. Perforation during colonoscopy in endoscopic ambulatory surgical centers. Gastrointest Endosc 2003;58(4):554–7.
10. Ko CW, Riffle S, Michaels L, et al. Serious complications within 30 days of screening and surveillance colonoscopy are uncommon. Clin Gastroenterol Hepatol 2010;8:166–73.
11. Ko CW, Riffle S, Shapiro JA, et al. Incidence of minor complications and time lost from normal activities after screening or surveillance colonoscopy. Gastrointest Endosc 2007;65(4):648–56.
12. Levin TR, Zhao W, Conell C, et al. Complications of colonoscopy in an integrated health care delivery system. Ann Intern Med 2006;145(12):880–6.
13. Rabeneck L, Paszat LF, Hilsden RJ, et al. Bleeding and perforation after outpatient colonoscopy and their risk factors in usual clinical practice. Gastroenterology 2008;135(6):1899–906.
14. Warren JL, Klabunde CN, Mariotto AB, et al. Adverse events after outpatient colonoscopy in the Medicare population. Ann Intern Med 2009;150(12):849–57.
15. Mandel JS, Bond JH, Church TR, et al. Reducing mortality from colorectal cancer by screening for fecal occult blood. N Engl J Med 1993;328:1365–71.
16. Zubarik R, Fleischer DE, Mastropietro C, et al. Prospective analysis of complications 30 days after outpatient colonoscopy. Gastrointest Endosc 1999;50(3):322–8.
17. Kewenter J, Brevinge H. Endoscopic and surgical complications of work-up in screening for colorectal cancer. Dis Colon Rectum 1996;39(6):676–80.

18. Tran DQ, Rosen L, Kim R, et al. Actual colonoscopy: what are the risks of perforation? Am Surg 2001;67(9):845–7 [discussion: 847–8].

19. Robinson MH, Hardcastle JD, Moss SM, et al. The risks of screening: data from the Nottingham randomised controlled trial of faecal occult blood screening for colorectal cancer. Gut 1999;45(4):588–92.

20. Thiis-Evensen E, Hoff GS, Sauar J, et al. Population-based surveillance by colonoscopy: effect on the incidence of colorectal cancer. Telemark Polyp Study I. Scand J Gastroenterol 1999;34(4):414–20.

21. Pickhardt PJ, Choi JR, Hwang I, et al. Computed tomographic virtual colonoscopy to screen for colorectal neoplasia in asymptomatic adults. N Engl J Med 2003;349(23):2191–200.

22. Segnan N, Senore C, Andreoni B, et al. Baseline findings of the Italian multicenter randomized controlled trial of "once-only sigmoidoscopy"—SCORE. J Natl Cancer Inst 2002;94(23):1763–72.

23. Cotterill M, Gasparelli R, Kirby E. Colorectal cancer detection in a rural community. Development of a colonoscopy screening program. Can Fam Physician 2005;51:1224–8.

24. Johnson CD, Chen MH, Toledano AY, et al. Accuracy of CT colonography for detection of large adenomas and cancers. N Engl J Med 2008;359(12):1207–17.

25. Rathgaber SW, Wick TM. Colonoscopy completion and complication rates in a community gastroenterology practice. Gastrointest Endosc 2006;64(4):556–62.

26. Farley DR, Bannon MP, Zietlow SP, et al. Management of colonoscopic perforations. Mayo Clin Proc 1997;72(8):729–33.

27. Iqbal CW, Chun YS, Farley DR. Colonoscopic perforations: a retrospective review. J Gastrointest Surg 2005;9(9):1229–35.

28. Luning TH, Keemers-Gels ME, Barendregt WB, et al. Colonoscopic perforations: a review of 30,366 patients. Surg Endosc 2007;21(6):994–7.

29. U.S. Preventive Services Task Force. Screening for colorectal cancer: U.S. Preventive Services Task Force recommendation statement. Ann Intern Med 2008;149(9):627–37.

30. Bini EJ, Firoozi B, Choung RJ, et al. Systematic evaluation of complications related to endoscopy in a training setting: a prospective 30-day outcomes study. Gastrointest Endosc 2003;57(1):8–16.

31. McQuaid KR, Laine L. A systematic review and meta-analysis of randomized, controlled trials of moderate sedation for routine endoscopic procedures. Gastrointest Endosc 2008;67(6):910–23.

32. Sharma VK, Nguyen CC, Crowell MD, et al. A national study of cardiopulmonary unplanned events after GI endoscopy. Gastrointest Endosc 2007;66(1):27–34.

33. Markowitz GS, Stokes MB, Radhakrishnan J, et al. Acute phosphate nephropathy following oral sodium phosphate bowel purgative: an underrecognized cause of chronic renal failure. J Am Soc Nephrol 2005;16(11):3389–96.

34. Markowitz GS, Radhakrishnan J, D'Agati VD. Towards the incidence of acute phosphate nephropathy. J Am Soc Nephrol 2007;18(12):3020–2.

35. Lieberman DA, Ghormley J, Flora K. Effect of oral sodium phosphate colon preparation on serum electrolytes in patients with normal serum creatinine. Gastrointest Endosc 1996;43(5):467–9.

36. Hurst FP, Bohen EM, Osgard EM, et al. Association of oral sodium phosphate purgative use with acute kidney injury. J Am Soc Nephrol 2007;18(12):3192–8.

37. Brunelli SM, Lewis JD, Gupta M, et al. Risk of kidney injury following oral phosphosoda bowel preparations. J Am Soc Nephrol 2007;18(12):3199–205.

38. Abaskharoun R, Depew W, Vanner S. Changes in renal function following administration of oral sodium phosphate or polyethylene glycol for colon cleansing before colonoscopy. Can J Gastroenterol 2007;21(4):227–31.
39. Singal AK, Rosman AS, Post JB, et al. The renal safety of bowel preparations for colonoscopy: a comparative study of oral sodium phosphate solution and polyethylene glycol. Aliment Pharmacol Ther 2008;27(1):41–7.
40. Food and Drug Administration. Oral sodium phosphate (OSP) products for bowel cleansing. Available at: http://www.fda.gov/Drugs/DrugSafety/PostmarketDrugSafetyInformationforPatientsandProviders/ucm103354.htm; 2008. Accessed January 28, 2010.
41. Wexner SD, Beck DE, Baron TH, et al. A consensus document on bowel preparation before colonoscopy: prepared by a task force from the American Society of Colon and Rectal Surgeons (ASCRS), the American Society for Gastrointestinal Endoscopy (ASGE), and the Society of American Gastrointestinal and Endoscopic Surgeons (SAGES). Gastrointest Endosc 2006;63(7):894–909.
42. Raymond PL. Mallory-Weiss tear associated with polyethylene glycol electrolyte lavage solution. Gastrointest Endosc 1991;37(3):410–1.
43. McBride MA, Vanagunas A. Esophageal perforation associated with polyethylene glycol electrolyte lavage solution. Gastrointest Endosc 1993;39(6):856–7.
44. Gabel A, Muller S. Aspiration: a possible severe complication in colonoscopy preparation of elderly people by orthograde intestine lavage. Digestion 1999;60(3):284–5.
45. Clark LE, Dipalma JA. Safety issues regarding colonic cleansing for diagnostic and surgical procedures. Drug Saf 2004;27(15):1235–42.
46. Nelson DB, Barkun AN, Block KP, et al. Technology status evaluation report. Colonoscopy preparations. Gastrointest Endosc 2001;54(6):829–32.
47. Ayus JC, Levine R, Arieff AI. Fatal dysnatraemia caused by elective colonoscopy. BMJ 2003;326(7385):382–4.
48. Rao KV, Beri GD, Sterling MJ, et al. Splenic injury as a complication of colonoscopy: a case series. Am J Gastroenterol 2009;104(6):1604–5.
49. Izzedine H, Thauvin H, Maisel A, et al. Post-colonoscopy appendicitis: case report and review of the literature. Am J Gastroenterol 2005;100(12):2815–7.
50. Chae HS, Kim SS, Han SW, et al. Herniation of the large bowel through a posttraumatic diaphragmatic defect during colonoscopy: report of a case. Dis Colon Rectum 2002;45(9):1261–2.
51. Bouma G, van Bodegraven AA, van Waesberghe JH, et al. Post-colonoscopy massive air leakage with full body involvement: an impressive complication with uneventful recovery. Am J Gastroenterol 2009;104(5):1330–2.
52. Jongwutiwes U, Shaukat A, Pocha C. Image of the month. Intramural cecal hematoma: a rare complication after colonoscopy. Clin Gastroenterol Hepatol 2009;7(7):A32.
53. Arhan M, Onal IK, Odemis B, et al. Colonoscopy-induced ischemic colitis in a young patient with no risk factor. Am J Gastroenterol 2009;104(1):250–1.
54. Bigard MA, Gaucher P, Lassalle C. Fatal colonic explosion during colonoscopic polypectomy. Gastroenterology 1979;77(6):1307–10.
55. Nelson DB. Infectious disease complications of GI endoscopy: Part I, endogenous infections. Gastrointest Endosc 2003;57(4):546–56.
56. Wilson W, Taubert KA, Gewitz M, et al. Prevention of infective endocarditis: guidelines from the American Heart Association: a guideline from the American Heart Association Rheumatic Fever, Endocarditis, and Kawasaki Disease Committee, Council on Cardiovascular Disease in the Young, and the Council on Clinical

Cardiology, Council on Cardiovascular Surgery and Anesthesia, and the Quality of Care and Outcomes Research Interdisciplinary Working Group. Circulation 2007;116(15):1736–54.

57. Banerjee S, Shen B, Baron TH, et al. Antibiotic prophylaxis for GI endoscopy. Gastrointest Endosc 2008;67(6):791–8.

58. Ahishali E, Uygur-Bayramicli O, Dolapcioglu C, et al. Chemical colitis due to Glutaraldehyde: case series and review of the literature. Dig Dis Sci 2009;54:2541–5.

59. Lee SK, Kim TI, Shin SJ, et al. Impact of prior abdominal or pelvic surgery on colonoscopy outcomes. J Clin Gastroenterol 2006;40(8):711–6.

60. Shah HA, Paszat LF, Saskin R, et al. Factors associated with incomplete colonoscopy: a population-based study. Gastroenterology 2007;132(7):2297–303.

61. Gilbert DA, DiMarino AJ, Jensen DM, et al. Status evaluation: hot biopsy forceps. American Society for Gastrointestinal Endoscopy. Technology Assessment Committee. Gastrointest Endosc 1992;38(6):753–6.

62. Dyer WS, Quigley EM, Noel SM, et al. Major colonic hemorrhage following electrocoagulating (hot) biopsy of diminutive colonic polyps: relationship to colonic location and low-dose aspirin therapy. Gastrointest Endosc 1991;37(3):361–4.

63. Weston AP, Campbell DR. Diminutive colonic polyps: histopathology, spatial distribution, concomitant significant lesions, and treatment complications. Am J Gastroenterol 1995;90(1):24–8.

64. Hui AJ, Wong RM, Ching JY, et al. Risk of colonoscopic polypectomy bleeding with anticoagulants and antiplatelet agents: analysis of 1657 cases. Gastrointest Endosc 2004;59(1):44–8.

65. Kim HS, Kim TI, Kim WH, et al. Risk factors for immediate postpolypectomy bleeding of the colon: a multicenter study. Am J Gastroenterol 2006;101(6): 1333–41.

66. Sawhney MS, Salfiti N, Nelson DB, et al. Risk factors for severe delayed postpolypectomy bleeding. Endoscopy 2008;40(2):115–9.

67. Shiffman ML, Farrel MT, Yee YS. Risk of bleeding after endoscopic biopsy or polypectomy in patients taking aspirin or other NSAIDS. Gastrointest Endosc 1994; 40(4):458–62.

68. Kwok A, Faigel DO. Management of anticoagulation before and after gastrointestinal endoscopy. Am J Gastroenterol 2009;104(12):3085–97.

69. Anderson MA, Ben-Menachem T, Gan SI, et al. Management of antithrombotic agents for endoscopic procedures. Gastrointest Endosc 2009;70(6): 1060–70.

70. Veitch AM, Baglin TP, Gershlick AH, et al. Guidelines for the management of anticoagulant and antiplatelet therapy in patients undergoing endoscopic procedures. Gut 2008;57(9):1322–9.

71. Church J, Delaney C. Randomized, controlled trial of carbon dioxide insufflation during colonoscopy. Dis Colon Rectum 2003;46(3):322–6.

72. Wong JC, Yau KK, Cheung HY, et al. Towards painless colonoscopy: a randomized controlled trial on carbon dioxide-insufflating colonoscopy. ANZ J Surg 2008;78(10):871–4.

73. Rex DK. Achieving cecal intubation in the very difficult colon. Gastrointest Endosc 2008;67(6):938–44.

74. Fatima H, Rex DK. Minimizing endoscopic complications: colonoscopic polypectomy. Gastrointest Endosc Clin N Am 2007;17(1):145–56, viii.

75. Panteris V, Haringsma J, Kuipers EJ. Colonoscopy perforation rate, mechanisms and outcome: from diagnostic to therapeutic colonoscopy. Endoscopy 2009; 41(11):941–51.

76. Lee SH, Lee KS, Park YS, et al. Submucosal saline-epinephrine injection in colon polypectomy: appropriate indication. Hepatogastroenterology 2008;55(86–87): 1589–93.

77. Iishi H, Tatsuta M, Iseki K, et al. Endoscopic piecemeal resection with submucosal saline injection of large sessile colorectal polyps. Gastrointest Endosc 2000;51(6):697–700.

78. Dobrowolski S, Dobosz M, Babicki A, et al. Prophylactic submucosal saline-adrenaline injection in colonoscopic polypectomy: prospective randomized study. Surg Endosc 2004;18(6):990–3.

79. Di Giorgio P, De Luca L, Calcagno G, et al. Detachable snare versus epinephrine injection in the prevention of postpolypectomy bleeding: a randomized and controlled study. Endoscopy 2004;36(10):860–3.

80. Paspatis GA, Paraskeva K, Theodoropoulou A, et al. A prospective, randomized comparison of adrenaline injection in combination with detachable snare versus adrenaline injection alone in the prevention of postpolypectomy bleeding in large colonic polyps. Am J Gastroenterol 2006;101(12):2805–9.

81. Parra-Blanco A, Kaminaga N, Kojima T, et al. Hemoclipping for postpolypectomy and postbiopsy colonic bleeding. Gastrointest Endosc 2000;51(1):37–41.

82. Lin CF, Cohen GS. Endoscopic repair of post-polypectomy colonic perforation. Am J Gastroenterol 2009;104(11):2869–70.

83. Ahlawat SK, Charabaty A, Benjamin S. Rectal perforation caused by retroflexion maneuver during colonoscopy: closure with endoscopic clips. Gastrointest Endosc 2008;67(4):771–3.

84. Institute of Medicine Committee on Quality of Health Care in America. To err is human: building a safer health system. Washington, DC: National Academies Press; 2000.

85. Gallagher TH, Waterman AD, Ebers AG, et al. Patients' and physicians' attitudes regarding the disclosure of medical errors. JAMA 2003;289(8):1001–7.

86. The Joint Commission. Hospital Accreditation Standards, 2007. Oakbrook Terrace (IL): Joint Commission Resources; 2007.

87. Gallagher TH. A 62-year-old woman with skin cancer who experienced wrong-site surgery: review of medical error. JAMA 2009;302(6):669–77.

88. Hasan AG, Brown WR. A model for mortality-morbidity conferences in gastroenterology. Gastrointest Endosc 2008;67(3):515–8.

89. Rex DK, Petrini JL, Baron TH, et al. Quality indicators for colonoscopy. Gastrointest Endosc 2006;63(Suppl 4):S16–28.

90. Dominitz JA, Ikenberry SO, Anderson MA, et al. Renewal of and proctoring for endoscopic privileges. Gastrointest Endosc 2008;67(1):10–6.

91. Department of Veterans Affairs Office of the Inspector General. Healthcare inspection: use and reprocessing of flexible fiberoptic endoscopes at VA medical facilities. Available at: http://www4.va.gov/oig/54/reports/VAOIG-09-01784-146. pdf; 2009. Accessed January 28, 2010.

92. American Society for Gastrointestinal Endoscopy. Multi-society guideline for reprocessing flexible gastrointestinal endoscopes. Gastrointest Endosc 2003; 58(1):1–8.

93. Banerjee S, Shen B, Nelson DB, et al. Infection control during GI endoscopy. Gastrointest Endosc 2008;67(6):781–90.

Efficacy and Effectiveness of Colonoscopy: How Do We Bridge the Gap?

David G. Hewett, MBBS, FRACP[a,b,*], Charles J. Kahi, MD, MSc[a],
Douglas K. Rex, MD[a]

KEYWORDS

- Colonoscopy • Efficacy • Effectiveness • Adenoma detection
- Colorectal cancer

Given that colorectal cancer (CRC) is the third leading cause of cancer death in the United States, its prevention is an important goal. Colonoscopy is sometimes considered the preferred CRC screening modality.[1] The primary goal of colonoscopy is the detection of colorectal adenomas and the prevention of CRC by interrupting the adenoma-carcinoma sequence. Evidence for the effectiveness of colonoscopy in reducing the incidence of CRC derives from observational studies and indirect evidence.[2] The performance of colonoscopy for this goal has been increasingly scrutinized with the publication of studies questioning its effectiveness, particularly in the proximal colon.[2–4]

Efficacy refers to the performance characteristics of a diagnostic test or any other medical intervention under ideal circumstances, whereas effectiveness refers to the performance characteristics of the test or intervention under usual circumstances in clinical practice.[5] Although a large number of quality indicators for the assessment of colonoscopy efficacy have been recommended[6,7] and CRC prevention is the ultimate goal of colonoscopy screening, adenoma detection is arguably the most important of all quality indicators[8] and represents an intermediate outcome in the spectrum of colorectal neoplasia. This article discusses issues in the efficacy-effectiveness concept as they relate to adenoma detection.

[a] Division of Gastroenterology, Department of Medicine, Indiana University School of Medicine, University Hospital 4100, 550 North University Boulevard, Indianapolis, IN 46202, USA
[b] School of Medicine, University of Queensland and Queensland Health Skills Development Centre, PO Box 470, Brisbane, Queensland 4029, Australia
* Corresponding author. Division of Gastroenterology, Department of Medicine, Indiana University School of Medicine, University Hospital 4100, 550 North University Boulevard, Indianapolis, IN 46202.
E-mail address: d.hewett@uq.edu.au

Gastrointest Endoscopy Clin N Am 20 (2010) 673–684
doi:10.1016/j.giec.2010.07.011
giendo.theclinics.com

THE EFFICACY OF COLONOSCOPY FOR ADENOMA DETECTION

Evidence for the efficacy of colonoscopy in detecting colorectal neoplasia derives from clinical trials of screening colonoscopy.[9–18] The polyp prevalence rates calculated from the trials in the United States conducted in asymptomatic, average-risk persons aged 50 years and older have yielded fairly consistent results, with mean adenoma prevalence ranging from 25% to 37%.[9–19] These prevalence rates have formed the basis of the current quality indicator thresholds for adenoma detection.[7]

However, in this article it is argued that the true efficacy of colonoscopy for adenoma detection has not been defined, while colonoscopy has been applied in routine clinical practice with suboptimal effectiveness for adenoma detection and CRC prevention. This argument is supported by increasing observational evidence that colonoscopy does not confer the high levels of protection against incident CRC that it was once thought it could.[2] Whereas early studies showed that colonoscopy and polypectomy prevent 76% to 90% of CRC,[20–22] data now suggest that the level of protection from colonoscopy may be only 50% or less,[23–25] with protection perhaps confined to the left colon.[2,3] Failures of colonoscopy to consistently detect adenomas or other precursors of CRC are therefore threatening the effectiveness of colonoscopy for the prevention of CRC.

Why is the true efficacy of colonoscopy undefined? First, studies of the efficacy of colonoscopy in detecting adenomas are limited by the lack of a criterion/gold standard against which the performance characteristics of the test can be evaluated. Second, most of the so-called efficacy studies were conducted in routine clinical academic or community practice, in which the testing conditions and participants were not necessarily optimized or standardized.[9–19] Therefore, these efficacy studies were subject to the same factors that influence the effectiveness of colonoscopy in clinical practice.

FACTORS LIMITING THE EFFECTIVENESS OF COLONOSCOPY

Limitations to the effectiveness of colonoscopy may be related to the patient, endoscopist, system, or technical factors (**Box 1**).[2] Patient factors include the quality of bowel preparation and tumor biology. Bowel preparation has been shown several times to contribute to polyp detection,[26–30] and the use of split-dose bowel preparations is now established as a critical element of quality colonoscopy.[30–39] Bowel preparation quality appears to be affected by socioeconomic status,[40] and lower levels of bowel preparation might contribute to the failure of colonoscopists serving indigent patients to achieve target thresholds. Tumor biology is also relevant, given the increasing recognition of flat lesions[41] and the serrated pathway of carcinogenesis.[42]

However, endoscopist-related operator dependency in colonoscopy performance is the major factor that threatens the effectiveness of colonoscopy in routine practice. Colonoscopy may be subject to operator dependency more than any other CRC prevention test. Many gastroenterologists have been documented to have adenoma detection rates less than the current targets.[43–46] The magnitude of within-group variation is substantial (4- to 10-fold) but is comparable when examined in academic,[43] mixed community-academic,[44] and community practices.[45,46] Differences in detection extend importantly to detection of large adenomas.[43,44] Given that colonoscopy plays a critical role in CRC prevention when it is used either for screening or for diagnosis with other positive screening tests and given the widespread acceptance of the importance of CRC prevention, the overall injury caused by suboptimal effectiveness of colonoscopy is substantial.

Box 1
Potential factors limiting the effectiveness of colonoscopy

Patient-related factors

- Poor bowel preparation
- Tumor biology (eg, genetic factors and environmental factors such as diet/smoking)

Colonoscopist-related factors

- Procedural/motor skill deficits (eg, incomplete colonoscopy, incomplete/inadequate polypectomy, and withdrawal technique)
- Perceptual factors (eg, variation in color and depth perception)
- Personality characteristics (conscientiousness, obsessiveness, and impulsivity)
- Knowledge and attitude deficits (eg, awareness and appearance of flat lesions)

System-related factors

- Financial factors (eg, reimbursement disincentives)
- Organizational factors (eg, workload pressures and level of training)

Technical factors

- Inadequate equipment (eg, poor image resolution)

Data from Hewett DG, Kahi CJ, Rex DK. Does colonoscopy work? J Natl Compr Canc Netw 2010;8(1):73; with permission.

Between-specialty variation has also been documented in colonoscopy performance. Primary care physicians performing colonoscopy have been shown several times to be more likely to miss CRC when compared with gastroenterologists,[47–49] and in Canada, performance of colonoscopy in the office setting is associated with an increased risk of missed cancer diagnosis.[50] These differences may reflect the differences in training in colonoscopy between primary care physicians and gastroenterologists. However, the purpose of developing quality targets for colonoscopy is to reduce variation in performance, that is, to bring all performance colonoscopy up to minimum accepted thresholds. Thus, although thresholds are derived from studies performed by gastroenterologists, quality targets derived from those studies are available for use and should be used by general surgeons and primary care physicians performing colonoscopy.

The potential negative effect of ineffective colonoscopy is apparent when considering the current postpolypectomy surveillance recommendations.[51] Postpolypectomy surveillance recommendations, by necessity, assume that the performance of colonoscopy is relatively uniform. In reality, the percentage of patients with one or more adenomas, with multiple adenomas, and with large adenomas differs substantially between endoscopists.[43,44] If endoscopists have low adenoma detection rates, they will incorrectly advise more adenoma-bearing patients that they are normal and can be followed up at 10 years, and more patients with 3 or more adenomas that they can be followed up at 5 years. Thus, a low-level adenoma detector following the current postpolypectomy surveillance recommendations would be expected to put a significant percentage of their patients at increased risk of an interval cancer. On the other hand, a high-level adenoma detector's patients are doubly protected. First, their patients' colons have been better cleared of adenomas at the baseline colonoscopy. Second, they are reassessing substantially more patients at 5 and 3 years' follow-up because of the presence of any adenoma, or of multiple (3 or more) adenomas and large adenomas respectively. Many colonoscopists do not follow post-polypectomy surveillance recommendations, perhaps because of lack of knowledge regarding the recommendations or lack of confidence in the recommendations.[52–55] Undoubtedly, many of these same colonoscopists have not measured their personal adenoma detection rates. Concern from endoscopists who have not measured their adenoma detection rate that current screening and surveillance recommendation intervals are too long is illogical and arguably irresponsible, because only a knowledge of the adenoma detection rate allows an estimate of whether an endoscopist is likely to be placing patients at risk for missed lesions.

Technical factors include the availability of quality endoscopic equipment, and system factors include those financial or organizational factors that may preclude or work against best practice. High-resolution white light colonoscopy has become widely available since the publication of adenoma detection targets, probably facilitating adenoma detection,[56–59] and therefore technology is unlikely to contribute to lower detection rates in clinical practice. Further technical innovations in colonoscopic imaging should make reaching adenoma detection targets even easier. In this regard, high-definition colonoscopy shows promise,[56–59] although other techniques such as pancolonic indigo carmine chromoendoscopy,[57] narrow band imaging,[56,60–64] and the Fuji Intelligent Chromo Endoscopy system (Fujinon Inc, Wayne, NJ, USA)[65] have generally yielded negative results regarding improvement in adenoma detection.

DEFINING THE TRUE EFFICACY OF COLONOSCOPY

Recommended thresholds for adenoma detection in asymptomatic persons aged 50 years and older are at present set at 25% for men and at 15% for women.[6,7] These targets were set by consideration of the mean prevalence rates of adenomas in screening colonoscopy studies. Thus, the mean adenoma prevalence rates in all screening colonoscopy studies in the United States have exceeded the recommended thresholds of 25% in men and 15% in women.[9–18] However, the same factors that limit the effectiveness of colonoscopy have also likely influenced the conduction of the original studies that have established the current definitions of the efficacy of colonoscopy.

In these studies, patient characteristics were not standardized. For example, the prevalence of adenomas is influenced not only by the age and gender of the study population[9–18] but also by additional factors such as the prevalence of smoking, obesity, diabetes, and a family history of CRC.[1] As a result, it is important to be cautious in generalizing the adenoma prevalence findings from these trials,[9–18] because there are insufficient data present to determine whether the study populations were typical of patients assessed in routine screening colonoscopy practice. However, because volunteers for studies are generally healthier than the general population, it is unlikely that differences between populations in clinical trials and clinical practice would result in practitioners being less likely to be able to achieve targeted neoplasia detection rates.[6,7] Other patient factors, such as the type and quality of bowel preparation, which have a clear influence on polyp detection, were not standardized in the efficacy studies. Split-dose preparations were not widely used at that time and tended to equalize differences in preparation quality between populations.[30–39]

Regarding endoscopist factors, the efficacy studies did not report variation in detection between the participating colonoscopists. However, there is every reason to think that the same level of variation between colonoscopists was present in these studies as has been found in other studies describing variable adenoma detection.[43–46] Technical factors are also likely to have influenced the measured efficacy in screening studies. Efficacy studies of screening colonoscopy are generally characterized by the use of white light endoscopy and standard-resolution colonoscopes, with high cecal intubation rates of 97% and more.[1]

Recent studies in which test conditions have been optimized have redefined the efficacy of colonoscopy for adenoma detection. These studies have shown that known high-level adenoma detectors using high-definition colonoscopes with high-quality bowel preparation find adenomas in 50% or more of the screening population. In most cases, the gain in adenoma detection is in diminutive and frequently in flat adenomas.[56–58] As a result, the costs and risks associated with removal of many diminutive adenomas assume increasing importance with increasing adenoma detection, and methods for real-time histologic assessment to allow small and diminutive adenomas to be "resected and discarded" are needed.[66,67]

Ultimately, these high rates of true adenoma prevalence could be used to increase adenoma detection targets. However, increasing targets raises the question of whether thresholds should be set at the arithmetical mean of all the studies, or perhaps the mean determined in a weighted fashion by the numbers of subjects in the studies, or at a different level, such as one-third (or 10%) of the mean adenoma prevalence rates in the studies. In this regard, the recommended adenoma detection thresholds are arbitrary. However, the current thresholds establish a cutoff level such that individuals with detection levels below the thresholds are definitely in the lowest half of adenoma detectors and are detecting less than half of those with adenomas. Given that many endoscopists have not yet measured their adenoma detection rates at all, it seems unnecessary to raise detection targets at this time, although this could be considered in the future.

In addition to variation in the documented prevalence rates of adenomas in screening colonoscopy, it is important to acknowledge the limitations of the adenoma detection rate as a definition of efficacy. The rate of adenoma detection in screening colonoscopy is only an intermediate outcome measure compared with the most definitive end-outcome measure, which is the incidence of interval cancer after clearing colonoscopy. Interval cancer incidence has been shown statistically to cluster within individual colonoscopists,[68] which would be expected given the current information about variable detection between endoscopists. However, adenoma detection is probably the best marker of the quality of mucosal inspection available.

Large adenoma detection is logically a superior outcome measure to overall adenoma detection, but is problematic to measure. The acceptable target thresholds for large adenoma detection are less clearly based on screening colonoscopy studies.[9–18] Second, measurement of the large-adenoma detection rate is more difficult because many more colonoscopies must be reviewed to determine the large-adenoma detection rate with narrow confidence intervals, simply because they are much less prevalent than adenomas in general. Third, the use of a large-adenoma detection rate introduces an error caused by endoscopic polyp size measurement. In addition, measurement bias could be introduced by endoscopists who simply designate polyps less than 1 cm in size as 1 cm or larger to reach the detection rate. Overall adenoma detection is not subject to this bias.

The best proposed alternative to the adenoma detection rate is the detection of number of adenomas per colonoscopy,[46,56,57] because it might best reflect the quality of mucosal examination over the entire length of the colon and have increased discriminatory power for good versus poor detectors. However, the best thresholds for number of adenomas detected per colonoscopy are not yet known. Thus, overall adenoma detection defined as a prevalence rate, that is, the percentage of patients aged 50 years and older with one or more adenomas, is likely to remain the single most important and feasible measure of colonoscopy efficacy. Overall adenoma detection has the advantage of being easy to measure and having been well studied in efficacy trials, and at least 2 studies show that it correlates with large adenoma detection.[43,46]

BRIDGING THE GAP: IMPROVING THE EFFECTIVENESS OF COLONOSCOPY

Interventions to improve the effectiveness of colonoscopy can operate at different levels within the health system[69] yet they need to target patient, endoscopist, technical, and system factors that affect quality.[2] Patient factors need to be optimized, including the use of modern bowel preparation methods such as split dosing. Other practice-level interventions to ensure high-quality preparations would be dependent on the patient population; practices serving indigent populations may need to use patient navigators[70,71] or even arrange for patients to complete bowel preparations in-facility. Technical factors should also be considered because the current thresholds are easy to meet if high-definition colonoscopes are used.[1,72]

For endoscopists, clearly the first step in bridging the gap between efficacy and effectiveness is to measure their adenoma detection rates as part of audit and feedback cycles within routine clinical practice. This performance measure, together with documentation of cecal intubation and other quality indicators,[7] should be incorporated into continuous quality improvement systems to allow local and national benchmarking of performance. Other system-level interventions that are worthy of consideration include payment reforms to align incentives with the value of colonoscopy performance.

Endoscopist factors that could underlie poor detection have not yet been investigated (see **Box 1**). Potential contributions include skill and knowledge deficits, visuo-perceptual factors, and personality characteristics.[2] Endoscopists with adenoma detection rates below threshold are clearly using inadequate mucosal inspection techniques. Deficits in skills and knowledge are potentially amenable to correction by training and credentialing processes, although inappropriate attitudes may be more resistant. Other endoscopist factors including visuoperceptual deficiencies and personality characteristics (such as risk taking and obsessiveness) deserve further evaluation, although these could be hard to address in established endoscopists. However, if clearly linked to detection, these factors could be incorporated into selection criteria for colonoscopy training programs.

Mucosal inspection techniques are not easily defined or assessed; however, low-level detectors typically perform colonoscopy rapidly and/or fail to visualize the colorectal mucosa because of inadequate fold examination, cleanup, and luminal distention.[73] Adenoma detection is associated with withdrawal time, although time is only one aspect of the range of inspection behaviors required for adenoma detection.[43–46,74]

The lack of definition regarding quality inspection technique limits the conduct of studies of interventions to correct poor performance in colonoscopy. In one study, the use of a timer that was targeted to 8 minutes' total withdrawal time and that sounded every 2 minutes improved adenoma detection across a range of endoscopists.[75] However, another trial with targeted withdrawal time gave negative results, emphasizing that withdrawal time may not be the behavior predictive of detection if the time is not spent actually searching for adenomas.[76] A series of interventions over several years in a large private practice group in Minnesota failed to improve low-level detectors.[45] Changing professional behavior is complex, and needs an understanding of the required behaviors and relevant theoretical frameworks to inform the design of effective quality improvement interventions.[77,78]

The extent to which inspection/withdrawal technique is taught in fellowship programs is uncertain, and without clear definitions of the component detection skills, training methods for developing high-level inspection competency are not well established. Adenoma detection, as an outcome indicator requiring a sufficient sample size for precise measurement,[79] is not necessarily appropriate for assessment of inspection competence during fellowship training. Hence, definitive validated methods of training and measuring mucosal inspection skill are required for use during colonoscopy training and for certification and recertification processes.

SUMMARY

Bridging the gap between the efficacy and effectiveness of colonoscopy entails reducing the variation in performance between endoscopists. Further, the very definition of efficacy in colonoscopy is problematic, because the original efficacy studies represent the results of a mean level of detection obtained from a group of colonoscopists who themselves have widely variable detection rates, even though all were considered well trained and expert. Prevalence rates from recent studies with known high-level adenoma detectors and optimized patient and technical factors are helping to define the true efficacy of colonoscopy. Current targets for adenoma detection appear to be broadly applicable to clinical practice and are easy to achieve. Hence, improvements in bowel preparation and advancements in colonoscopy should make current thresholds easier rather than more difficult to achieve. However, similarities between the efficacy and effectiveness studies with regard to both overall adenoma prevalence rates and variable detection by endoscopists suggest that more- and less-effective endoscopists are part of virtually every group of endoscopists. Substantial variations in performance exist not only between specialties but also within members of the same specialty who have received similar training. Thus, correcting within-group variation in both academic and community practices may be the central performance issue in colonoscopy.

The gap between efficacy and effectiveness for adenoma detection mirrors the evidence-practice gap seen in many other areas of health care.[80] Interventions to motivate change in physician behavior are required to improve adenoma detection by low-level detectors, which should be targeted at various levels in the health system. Research is required to define the necessary mucosal inspection skills and training required for high-level adenoma detectors. Colonoscopy should now be performed only in the context of quality measurement, which is the key to defining the extent of variable performance and developing systems for ensuring value-based colonoscopy.

REFERENCES

1. Rex DK, Johnson DA, Anderson JC, et al. American College of Gastroenterology guidelines for colorectal cancer screening 2009. Am J Gastroenterol 2009;104(3): 739–50.
2. Hewett DG, Kahi CJ, Rex DK. Does colonoscopy work? J Natl Compr Canc Netw 2010;8(1):67–77.
3. Brenner H, Hoffmeister M, Arndt V, et al. Protection from right- and left-sided colorectal neoplasms after colonoscopy: population-based study. J Natl Cancer Inst 2010;102(2):89–95.

4. Baxter NN, Rabeneck L. Is the effectiveness of colonoscopy "good enough" for population-based screening? J Natl Cancer Inst 2010;102(2):70–1.
5. Haynes RB, Sackett DL, Guyatt GH, et al. Clinical epidemiology: how to do clinical practice research. 3rd edition. Philadelphia: Lippincott Williams & Wilkins; 2006.
6. Rex DK, Bond JH, Winawer S, et al. Quality in the technical performance of colonoscopy and the continuous quality improvement process for colonoscopy: recommendations of the U.S. Multi-Society Task Force on Colorectal Cancer. Am J Gastroenterol 2002;97(6):1296–308.
7. Rex DK, Petrini JL, Baron TH, et al. Quality indicators for colonoscopy. Am J Gastroenterol 2006;101(4):873–85.
8. Rex DK. Who is the best colonoscopist? Gastrointest Endosc 2007;65(1):145–50.
9. Johnson DA, Gurney MS, Volpe RJ, et al. A prospective study of the prevalence of colonic neoplasms in asymptomatic patients with an age-related risk. Am J Gastroenterol 1990;85(8):969–74.
10. Foutch PG, Mai H, Pardy K, et al. Flexible sigmoidoscopy may be ineffective for secondary prevention of colorectal cancer in asymptomatic, average-risk men. Dig Dis Sci 1991;36(7):924–8.
11. Lieberman DA, Smith FW. Screening for colon malignancy with colonoscopy. Am J Gastroenterol 1991;86(8):946–51.
12. Rogge JD, Elmore MF, Mahoney SJ, et al. Low-cost, office-based, screening colonoscopy. Am J Gastroenterol 1994;89(10):1775–80.
13. Rex D, Sledge G, Harper P, et al. Colonic neoplasia in asymptomatic persons with negative fecal occult blood tests: influence of age, gender, and family history. Am J Gastroenterol 1993;88:825–31.
14. Kadakia SC, Wrobleski CS, Kadakia AS, et al. Prevalence of proximal colonic polyps in average-risk asymptomatic patients with negative fecal occult blood tests and flexible sigmoidoscopy. Gastrointest Endosc 1996;44(2):112–7.
15. Lieberman DA, Weiss DG, Bond JH, et al. Use of colonoscopy to screen asymptomatic adults for colorectal cancer. N Engl J Med 2000;343(3):162–8.
16. Imperiale T, Wagner D, Lin C, et al. Risk of advanced proximal neoplasms in asymptomatic adults according to the distal colorectal findings. N Engl J Med 2000;343:169–74.
17. Imperiale TF, Ransohoff DF, Itzkowitz SH, et al. Fecal DNA versus fecal occult blood for colorectal-cancer screening in an average-risk population. N Engl J Med 2004;351(26):2704–14.
18. Schoenfeld P, Cash B, Flood A, et al. Colonoscopic screening of average-risk women for colorectal neoplasia. N Engl J Med 2005;352(20):2061–8.
19. Regula J, Rupinski M, Kraszewska E, et al. Colonoscopy in colorectal-cancer screening for detection of advanced neoplasia. N Engl J Med 2006;355(18):1863–72.
20. Winawer SJ, Zauber AG, Ho MN, et al. Prevention of colorectal cancer by colonoscopic polypectomy. N Engl J Med 1993;329(27):1977–81.
21. Citarda F, Tomaselli G, Capocaccia R, et al. Efficacy in standard clinical practice of colonoscopic polypectomy in reducing colorectal cancer incidence. Gut 2001; 48:812–5.
22. Thiis-Evensen E, Hoff G, Sauar J, et al. Population-based surveillance by colonoscopy: effect on the incidence of colorectal cancer. Telemark Polyp Study I. Scand J Gastroenterol 1999;34:414–20.
23. Schatzkin A, Lanza E, Corle D, et al. Lack of effect of a low-fat, high-fiber diet on the recurrence of colorectal adenomas. N Engl J Med 2000;342(16):1149–55.

24. Alberts DS, Martinez ME, Roe DJ, et al. Lack of effect of a high-fiber cereal supplement on the recurrence of colorectal adenomas. N Engl J Med 2000; 342(16):1156–62.
25. Robertson DJ, Greenberg ER, Beach M, et al. Colorectal cancer in patients under close colonoscopic surveillance. Gastroenterology 2005;129(1):34–41.
26. Harewood GC, Sharma VK, de Garmo P. Impact of colonoscopy preparation quality on detection of suspected colonic neoplasia. Gastrointest Endosc 2003; 58(1):76–9.
27. Froehlich F, Wietlisbach V, Gonvers JJ, et al. Impact of colonic cleansing on quality and diagnostic yield of colonoscopy: the European Panel of Appropriateness of Gastrointestinal Endoscopy European multicenter study. Gastrointest Endosc 2005;61(3):378–84.
28. Jain S, Johnson WD, Minocha A. Impact of quality of bowel preparation on the detection of colonic polyps during colonoscopy: a prospective study. Gastroenterology 2007;132:A315.
29. Cohen L, Kastenberg D, Lottes SR, et al. Polyp detection rate during colonoscopy is correlated with quality of bowel preparation. Am J Gastroenterol 2006; 101:S556.
30. Parra-Blanco A, Nicolas-Perez D, Gimeno-Garcia A, et al. The timing of bowel preparation before colonoscopy determines the quality of cleansing, and is a significant factor contributing to the detection of flat lesions: a randomized study. World J Gastroenterol 2006;12(38):6161–6.
31. Rostom A, Jolicoeur E, Dube C, et al. A randomized prospective trial comparing different regimens of oral sodium phosphate and polyethylene glycol-based lavage solution in the preparation of patients for colonoscopy. Gastrointest Endosc 2006;64(4):544–52.
32. Aoun E, Abdul-Baki H, Azar C, et al. A randomized single-blind trial of split-dose PEG-electrolyte solution without dietary restriction compared with whole dose PEG-electrolyte solution with dietary restriction for colonoscopy preparation. Gastrointest Endosc 2005;62(2):213–8.
33. Park JS, Sohn CI, Hwang SJ, et al. Quality and effect of single dose versus split dose of polyethylene glycol bowel preparation for early-morning colonoscopy. Endoscopy 2007;39(7):616–9.
34. Church JM. Effectiveness of polyethylene glycol antegrade gut lavage bowel preparation for colonoscopy—timing is the key! Dis Colon Rectum 1998;41(10): 1223–5.
35. El Sayed AM, Kanafani ZA, Mourad FH, et al. A randomized single-blind trial of whole versus split-dose polyethylene glycol-electrolyte solution for colonoscopy preparation. Gastrointest Endosc 2003;58(1):36–40.
36. Frommer D. Cleansing ability and tolerance of three bowel preparations for colonoscopy. Dis Colon Rectum 1997;40(1):100–4.
37. Abdul-Baki H, Hashash JG, Elhajj II, et al. A randomized, controlled, double-blind trial of the adjunct use of tegaserod in whole-dose or split-dose polyethylene glycol electrolyte solution for colonoscopy preparation. Gastrointest Endosc 2008;68(2):294–300 [quiz: 334, 336].
38. Chiu HM, Lin JT, Wang HP, et al. The impact of colon preparation timing on colonoscopic detection of colorectal neoplasms—a prospective endoscopist-blinded randomized trial. Am J Gastroenterol 2006;101(12):2719–25.
39. Gupta T, Mandot A, Desai D, et al. Comparison of two schedules (previous evening versus same morning) of bowel preparation for colonoscopy. Endoscopy 2007;39(8):706–9.

40. Rex DK, Imperiale TF, Latinovich DR, et al. Impact of bowel preparation on efficiency and cost of colonoscopy. Am J Gastroenterol 2002;97(7):1696–700.
41. Soetikno RM, Kaltenbach T, Rouse RV, et al. Prevalence of nonpolypoid (flat and depressed) colorectal neoplasms in asymptomatic and symptomatic adults. JAMA 2008;299(9):1027–35.
42. Leggett B, Whitehall V. Role of the serrated pathway in colorectal cancer pathogenesis. Gastroenterology 2010;138:2088–100.
43. Chen SC, Rex DK. Endoscopist can be more powerful than age and male gender in predicting adenoma detection at colonoscopy. Am J Gastroenterol 2007; 102(4):856–61.
44. Imperiale TF, Glowinski EA, Juliar BE, et al. Variation in polyp detection rates at screening colonoscopy. Gastrointest Endosc 2009;69(7):1288–95.
45. Shaukat A, Oancea C, Bond JH, et al. Variation in detection of adenomas and polyps by colonoscopy and change over time with a performance improvement program. Clin Gastroenterol Hepatol 2009;7(12):1335–40.
46. Barclay RL, Vicari JJ, Doughty AS, et al. Colonoscopic withdrawal times and adenoma detection during screening colonoscopy. N Engl J Med 2006; 355(24):2533–41.
47. Rex DK, Rahmani EY, Haseman JH, et al. Relative sensitivity of colonoscopy and barium enema for detection of colorectal cancer in clinical practice. Gastroenterology 1997;112(1):17–23.
48. Bressler B, Paszat LF, Vinden C, et al. Colonoscopic miss rates for right-sided colon cancer: a population-based analysis. Gastroenterology 2004;127(2):452–6.
49. Singh H, Turner D, Xue L, et al. Risk of developing colorectal cancer following a negative colonoscopy examination: evidence for a 10-year interval between colonoscopies. JAMA 2006;295(20):2366–73.
50. Bressler B, Paszat LF, Chen Z, et al. Rates of new or missed colorectal cancers after colonoscopy and their risk factors: a population-based analysis. Gastroenterology 2007;132(1):96–102.
51. Winawer SJ, Zauber AG, Fletcher RH, et al. Guidelines for colonoscopy surveillance after polypectomy: a consensus update by the US Multi-Society Task Force on Colorectal Cancer and the American Cancer Society. Gastroenterology 2006; 130(6):1872–85.
52. Mysliwiec PA, Brown ML, Klabunde CN, et al. Are physicians doing too much colonoscopy? A national survey of colorectal surveillance after polypectomy. Ann Intern Med 2004;141(4):264–71.
53. Burke C, Issa M, Church J. A nationwide survey of post-polypectomy surveillance colonoscopy: too many too soon! Gastroenterology 2005;128:A566.
54. Saini SD, Nayak RS, Kuhn L, et al. Why don't gastroenterologists follow colon polyp surveillance guidelines? Results of a national survey. J Clin Gastroenterol 2009;43(6):554–8.
55. Schoen RE, Pinsky PF, Weissfeld JL, et al. Utilization of surveillance colonoscopy in community practice. Gastroenterology 2010;138:73–81.
56. Rex DK, Helbig CC. High yields of small and flat adenomas with high-definition colonoscopes using either white light or narrow band imaging. Gastroenterology 2007;133(1):42–7.
57. Kahi C, Anderson J, Waxman I, et al. High-definition chromocolonoscopy versus high-definition white light colonoscopy for average-risk colorectal cancer screening. Am J Gastroenterol 2010;105(6):1301–7.
58. East JE, Stavrindis M, Thomas-Gibson S, et al. A comparative study of standard vs. high definition colonoscopy for adenoma and hyperplastic polyp detection

with optimized withdrawal technique. Aliment Pharmacol Ther 2008;28(6): 768–76.

59. Buchner AM, Shahid MW, Heckman MG, et al. High-definition colonoscopy detects colorectal polyps at a higher rate than standard white-light colonoscopy. Clin Gastroenterol Hepatol 2010;8(4):364–70.

60. Adler A, Pohl H, Papanikolaou IS, et al. A prospective randomised study on narrow-band imaging versus conventional colonoscopy for adenoma detection: does narrow-band imaging induce a learning effect? Gut 2008;57(1):59–64.

61. Adler A, Aschenbeck J, Yenerim T, et al. Narrow-band versus white-light high definition television endoscopic imaging for screening colonoscopy: a prospective randomized trial. Gastroenterology 2009;136(2):410–6, e411 [quiz: 715].

62. Kaltenbach T, Friedland S, Soetikno R. A randomised tandem colonoscopy trial of narrow band imaging versus white light examination to compare neoplasia miss rates. Gut 2008;57(10):1406–12.

63. Inoue T, Murano M, Murano N, et al. Comparative study of conventional colonoscopy and pan-colonic narrow-band imaging system in the detection of neoplastic colonic polyps: a randomized, controlled trial. J Gastroenterol 2008;43(1):45–50.

64. Paggi S, Radaelli F, Amato A, et al. The impact of narrow band imaging in screening colonoscopy: a randomized controlled trial. Clin Gastroenterol Hepatol 2009;7(10):1049–54.

65. Togashi K, Osawa H, Koinuma K, et al. A comparison of conventional endoscopy, chromoendoscopy, and the optimal-band imaging system for the differentiation of neoplastic and non-neoplastic colonic polyps. Gastrointest Endosc 2009;69(Suppl 3):734–41.

66. Ignjatovic A, East JE, Suzuki N, et al. Optical diagnosis of small colorectal polyps at routine colonoscopy (Detect InSpect ChAracterise Resect and Discard; DISCARD trial): a prospective cohort study. Lancet Oncol 2009;10(12):1171–8.

67. Rex DK. Narrow-band imaging without optical magnification for histologic analysis of colorectal polyps. Gastroenterology 2009;136(4):1174–81.

68. Gupta R, Brownlow B, Domnick R, et al. Colon cancer not prevented by colonoscopy. Am J Gastroenterol 2008;103(S1):S551.

69. Ferlie EB, Shortell SM. Improving the quality of health care in the United Kingdom and the United States: a framework for change. Milbank Q 2001;79(2):281–315.

70. Kazarian ES, Carreira FS, Toribara NW, et al. Colonoscopy completion in a large safety net health care system. Clin Gastroenterol Hepatol 2008;6(4):438–42.

71. Chen LA, Santos S, Jandorf L, et al. A program to enhance completion of screening colonoscopy among urban minorities. Clin Gastroenterol Hepatol 2008;6(4):443–50.

72. Rex DK. Maximizing detection of adenomas and cancers during colonoscopy. Am J Gastroenterol 2006;101(12):2866–77.

73. Rex DK. Colonoscopic withdrawal technique is associated with adenoma miss rates. Gastrointest Endosc 2000;51(1):33–6.

74. Simmons DT, Harewood GC, Baron TH, et al. Impact of endoscopist withdrawal speed on polyp yield: implications for optimal colonoscopy withdrawal time. Aliment Pharmacol Ther 2006;24(6):965–71.

75. Barclay RL, Vicari JJ, Greenlaw RL. Effect of a time-dependent colonoscopic withdrawal protocol on adenoma detection during screening colonoscopy. Clin Gastroenterol Hepatol 2008;6(10):1091–8.

76. Sawhney MS, Cury MS, Neeman N, et al. Effect of institution-wide policy of colonoscopy withdrawal time > or = 7 minutes on polyp detection. Gastroenterology 2008;135(6):1892–8.

77. Michie S, Johnston M, Abraham C, et al. Making psychological theory useful for implementing evidence based practice: a consensus approach. Qual Saf Health Care 2005;14(1):26–33.

78. Eccles M, Grimshaw J, Walker A, et al. Changing the behavior of healthcare professionals: the use of theory in promoting the uptake of research findings. J Clin Epidemiol 2005;58(2):107–12.

79. Dimick JB, Welch HG, Birkmeyer JD. Surgical mortality as an indicator of hospital quality: the problem with small sample size. JAMA 2004;292(7):847–51.

80. Institute of Medicine. Crossing the quality chasm: a new health system for the 21st century. Washington, DC: National Academies Press; 2001.

Colonoscopy Reports and Current State of Performance Measures

Jason E. Williams, MD, MPH, Douglas O. Faigel, MD*

KEYWORDS

• Colonoscopy • Quality • Performance • Measures

Documentation and measurement are essential to the Plan-Do-Study-Act model commonly used for quality improvement projects. Consequently, colonoscopy reports and performance measures are crucial to quality improvement programs and efforts aimed at maximizing the value of colonoscopy. In the past, however, colonoscopy reports garnered very little attention, and few measures of colonoscopy quality were endorsed. A growth in interest in colonoscopy quality has been paralleled with a growth in interest in these topics. Recently, societies and task forces have begun to advocate for standardized colonoscopy reports and to identify key performance measures (also known as *quality indicators*) for colonoscopy.[1–3] The use of precise and comprehensive colonoscopy reports and the regular assessment of quality indicators may lead to several rewards, including better patient outcomes, fewer complications, improved coordination of care, greater patient satisfaction, and improved reimbursement.

COLONOSCOPY REPORTS
Role

Colonoscopy reports serve various different functions and are used by various different parties. First and foremost, the colonoscopy report is a clinical document. For the referring provider and other clinicians, the report renders diagnoses and recommended therapies, and the timing and interval for future examinations. The report may also help endoscopists prepare for future examinations through providing critical information about sedation and instrument requirements, response to bowel cleansing strategies, patient tolerance, and any complications. Second, the colonoscopy report can be used for quality assurance and improvement processes. Quality measurement

The authors have nothing to disclose.
Division of Gastroenterology and Hepatology, Department of Medicine, Oregon Health and Science University, 3181 SW Sam Jackson Park Road (L-461), Portland, OR, USA
* Corresponding author.
E-mail address: faigeld@ohsu.edu

Gastrointest Endoscopy Clin N Am 20 (2010) 685–697
doi:10.1016/j.giec.2010.07.006
1052-5157/10/$ – see front matter © 2010 Elsevier Inc. All rights reserved.

information may be obtained, such as cecal intubation, quality of the preparation, and withdrawal time. Third, the colonoscopy report may have medicolegal implications. Fourth, colonoscopy reports are important for reimbursement. Inaccurate documentation of procedure indications or techniques used might translate into more time and effort spent obtaining reimbursement from payers.

Current State

Only a few studies have rigorously examined the quality of endoscopy reports, and most have shown incomplete reporting for several items.[4–6] Robertson and colleagues[5] examined reports from 122 endoscopy centers and found a substantial proportion of reports were missing key data, such as bowel preparation adequacy (70.5%), complications (41.8%), polyp size (26.2%), postprocedure recommendations (31.1%), sedation dose (27.1%), patient history (42.5%), and demographics (30.4%). More recently, Lieberman and colleagues[6] queried 438,521 colonoscopy reports and also found that many were missing key data, including bowel preparation quality (13.9%), comorbidity classification (10.1%), description of cecal landmarks (14.7%), and polyp size (4.9%). Across practices, significant variation was seen in the inclusion of certain elements. For instance, the bowel preparation quality was missing in more than 20% of procedures at 14 of the 52 endoscopy centers. In another recent study, only 33.5% of reports included follow-up recommendations.[7]

Colonoscopy Reporting and Data System

Recognizing that the absence of comprehensive and standardized colonoscopy reports has actually impeded quality measurement for colonoscopy, the Quality Assurance Task Group of the National Colorectal Cancer Roundtable developed the colonoscopy reporting and data system (CO-RADS) in 2007.[3] The group modeled CO-RADS after work performed to standardize the reporting of other screening tests (mammography and CT colonography) and was developed with the expertise of individuals in gastroenterology, radiology, primary care, and health care delivery. The group had the goal of creating a system that included a colonoscopy report with standardized elements and terminology that would allow measurement of quality within and across practices. For each of the following items, CO-RADS identifies important subitems that should be specifically addressed.

Elements of a Quality Report

Patient demographics and history: age, gender, anticoagulation management plan, presence of intraventricular defibrillator device or pacemaker (and management plan)

Certain patient characteristics have a significant impact on the yield and safety of colonoscopy. The age and gender of a patient affect the risk of finding adenomas or colorectal cancer.[8,9] Patients who require chronic anticoagulation or have implantable defibrillators or pacemakers are at higher risk for certain complications and deserve special attention. Other important preprocedure data includes documentation of informed consent and the type of facility where the colonoscopy is performed (eg, hospital, ambulatory surgery center or office).

Assessment of patient risk and comorbidity: American Society of Anesthesiologists classification

The American Society of Anesthesiologists (ASA) classification is one of the most commonly used risk assessment tools for colonoscopy. Although variability may exist between providers, the ASA has been used to predict perioperative mortality for many years and has been embraced by numerous specialties as a useful aid in measuring patient comorbidity. Furthermore, researchers have shown an association between preprocedure risk class and the rate of adverse events.[10] Assessing a patient's risk for complications is a process that may guide decisions regarding procedure setting, staff, and specific precautions.

Indications

Information about previous colonoscopies, along with risk factors, past medical history, and symptoms, help determine if and when a colonoscopy should be performed. Documentation of indications also provides a context for the procedure and explains why certain aspects of the procedure are performed or avoided (eg, not removing a tiny polyp during a procedure to treat hematochezia). This information should include information on the following:

- All indications: date of last colonoscopy, family history of colorectal cancer, adenomas, inherited syndrome
- Surveillance examinations: most advanced previous lesion, extent of last examination, adequacy of last bowel preparation
- Inflammatory bowel disease (IBD) surveillance: duration, extent, activity of disease; date of last examination; biopsy protocol used.

Procedure

Technical descriptions regarding the procedure should be documented, such as:

- Date and time
- Sedation: type, dose, provider responsible for sedation, level of sedation
- Extent of examination, reason incomplete (if applicable), method of verifying extent
- Time of examination: time when colonoscope inserted into rectum, when withdrawal from cecum started, when colonoscope was withdrawn from patient
- Performance of retroflexion
- Bowel preparation: type, dose, quality (adequacy to detect polyps >5 mm)
- Performance: difficulty, patient tolerance, special maneuvers
- Type of instrument: model and instrument number (could be reported in nursing record).

Bowel preparation has been shown to influence the sensitivity of colonoscopy for neoplasia detection.[11,12] Furthermore, the quality of bowel preparation then influences the timing for surveillance examinations. Recognizing that qualitative assessments can be subjective, CO-RADS authors advocate a more objective assessment similar to that used in the field of CT-colonography: adequacy to detect lesions greater than 5 mm. Reaching the cecum and documenting cecal anatomy are important steps, because a substantial number of advanced adenomas and cancers are found in the proximal colon.[13] Without information about the extent of the examination, whether the patient needs additional testing is unclear.

Several studies have shown an association between withdrawal time and detection of neoplastic lesions, but several caveats remain. The optimal withdrawal time is unknown; one group of authors investigated a 6-minute threshold and found a linear relationship between withdrawal time and adenoma detection (ADR), with no plateau in ADR.[14] However, in another study, longer withdrawal time was not associated with higher rates of neoplasia detection.[15] Although both the CO-RADS authors and the American Society for Gastrointestinal Endoscopy/American College of Gastroenterology (ASGE/ACG) Task Force on Quality in Endoscopy endorse measurement of withdrawal, the ASGE/ACG Task Force recommends measurement of withdrawal time primarily in settings of low adenoma detection. Whether withdrawal time should be documented on the colonoscopy report is not without controversy. A "short" withdrawal time on an individual report may lead to confusion because it may erroneously lead one to believe that the quality of a specific examination was suboptimal. Withdrawal times only have meaning when looked at in aggregate, as a mean, and as part of a quality assurance program.

The amount and type of sedation, patient tolerance, and overall difficulty of the examination may help in planning for future examinations. Instrument details must be recorded (either in the report or nursing records) to allow endoscope tracking if infection transmission is a concern.

Colonoscopic findings

Colonoscopic findings should be reported, including:

- Masses: location, size (in millimeters or centimeters), descriptors, biopsy, tattoo
- Polyps: location, size, morphology, biopsy or removal method, removal completion, retrieval, whether sent to pathology, tattoo
- Polyp cluster: same as for polyps, plus number in segment
- Submucosal lesions: same as for polyps
- Mucosal abnormality: suspected diagnosis, location, pathology obtained
- Other: diverticulosis, arteriovenous malformations, hemorrhoids, description of mucosa and whether biopsy performed in patients with diarrhea.

The effectiveness of colonoscopy for colorectal cancer screening depends on the identification and appropriate management of neoplastic lesions. The specific characteristics of a lesion influence the risk of recurrent lesions and are the basis of recommendations regarding the timing of future examinations. One particular polyp descriptor that was mentioned was the polyp size. Size plays a key role in determining intervals and size should be described in terms of millimeters, rather than vague qualitative terms.

Assessment

Impressions based on symptoms, laboratory studies, radiographic studies, and colonoscopic findings should be included in the report.

The assessment section of a colonoscopy report should incorporate clinical data from the colonoscopy within the context of the available data from the history and physical, laboratory values, and radiographic studies. Aside from these basic parameters, the CO-RADS group did not propose specific guidelines on the composition of the assessment section.

Interventions/unplanned events

Both immediate and delayed events/interventions should be recorded, including the type of event and the intervention used. Immediate events and interventions are obviously more easily recognized and reported, but delayed events (within 30 days) are also important, and include unplanned health visits or emergency department visits, hospitalization, blood transfusions, surgery, and death (including cause). Despite the difficulty, unplanned events should still be studied, and is easier when reports include complete and accurate information.

Follow-up plan

Various diagnostic and therapeutic recommendations may be made after colonoscopy. Patients only retain a fraction of medical information in medical encounters, and this fraction is likely to be less after administration of sedatives during colonoscopy. The colonoscopy report can relay important messages to referring physicians and help preserve continuity of care when it includes items such as:

- Future tests, referrals, medication changes, appointments
- Interval for follow-up colonoscopy (reason for nonguideline intervention)
- No further fecal occult blood testing for ≥ 5 years
- Communication to the patient and referring provider.

Pathology

A substantial proportion of colonoscopies include pathology specimens. Along with gross polyp descriptors, pathology of specimens also dramatically affect the timing of future examinations. Results should be reviewed and communicated to the referring provider and patient, along with a follow-up plan.

PERFORMANCE MEASURES
Defining and Measuring Quality

According to one industry survey, almost 90% of gastroenterologists already collect quality information or intend to do so soon.[16] Assessment of quality and performance measures (or quality indicators), however, depends on how one defines quality. Health care professionals have traditionally defined quality in terms of the technical excellence of medical care and the nature of provider–patient interactions.[17] Technical excellence consists of two aspects: the appropriateness of care and the skill with which care is provided. In essence, it is "doing the right thing right."[17] The nature of provider–patient interactions depends on clear communication, trust, concern, and sensitivity.

Although quality can be defined in various ways, quality measures have only three basic types: structure, process, and outcomes.[18,19] Structure deals with the organizational infrastructure, including the facility and provider characteristics (eg, physician training and specialty). Processes are the components of care or steps taken by a provider to achieve some end point (eg, performing random biopsies for chronic diarrhea). Finally, outcomes refer to health status and are the result of structure and processes (eg, colonic perforation or adenoma detection).

Process Measures

Several features make process measures appealing. First, process measures are often clearly defined and simple, making them easier to measure than outcomes. Second, unlike outcome measures, process measures typically do not need to be adjusted for differences in patient characteristics. Third, when a good process measure is identified, it highlights a specific action or technique on which a provider can focus to improve health outcomes. Fourth, process measures are often more sensitive than outcome measures.

For example, two endoscopists may have dramatically different rates of cecal intubation but very similar rates of colon cancer detection. As this example illustrates, an outcome measure sometimes will not detect poor quality care even when poor quality care occurs. This scenario is more common when certain outcomes (eg, colon cancer detection) are relatively infrequent and a large number of encounters are required to calculate reliable estimates for their frequency.

Process measures also have limitations; they often have no intrinsic worth. A process measure is only useful if a clear link exists between the process and a clinically relevant outcome. Process measures face a test of validity and are not always accepted as meaningful by patients, providers, or payers. Additionally, individual process measures usually only assess one specific element of care, but do not yield a comprehensive evaluation of care.

Outcome Measures

Outcomes are more intuitive measures; they typically do have intrinsic worth and are often the purpose for the health care processes. These measures usually matter most to individual patients and purchasers of care. One of the major limitations of outcomes measures is the fact that patient characteristics can profoundly affect health outcomes. Thus, comparison of outcome measures across providers or groups often requires risk adjustment to ensure that differences in patient populations can be accounted for and valid comparisons can be made. For instance, adenoma detection can be influenced by age, gender, and quality of bowel preparation, among other things.

Because outcome measures are influenced by several factors other than a provider's actions, providers will often have some degree of concern about the validity of outcome measures. Additionally, although health outcomes are the ultimate goal of care, measuring outcomes does not always provide physicians with specific targetable actions or steps they can address to improve. Also, certain outcomes are rare or a substantial delay occurs between care and health outcomes. For colonoscopy, perforations and colorectal cancers are too rare to offer meaningful comparisons until large sample sizes are amassed. Finally, although processes can often be collected easily during routine clinical care, outcomes data analysis often requires additional steps outside of the clinical encounter.

Ideal Measures

Rising health care costs and an emphasis on quality improvement have spurred discussion about characteristics of ideal quality measures across medicine, including gastroenterology.[20–22] Colonoscopy quality measures are considered desirable if they are closely linked to relevant outcomes, evidence-based, auditable, easily integrated into practice, aimed at quality improvement (not cost-containment), and developed by a consensus process involving gastroenterology societies. Ideal measures should also be resistant to unintended consequences, and collection of measures should not be overly time-consuming. In 2006, the ASGE and the ACG formed the ASGE/ACG Task Force on Quality in Endoscopy and proposed a list of quality indicators for colonoscopy.[1] These indicators are applied to three periods: preprocedure, which encompasses all contacts with the patient until sedation or scope insertion; intraprocedure, which encompasses scope insertion through withdrawal; and postprocedure, which encompasses recovery through follow-up.

Quality Measures for Colonoscopy

Preprocedure
Indication The indication for colonoscopy should be documented and consistent with ASGE and U.S. Multi-Society Task Force on Colon Cancer indications. If a nonstandard indication is used, the rationale for this decision should be included.

When endoscopists perform colonoscopy for appropriate indications, they are more likely to make clinically relevant diagnoses.[23] Still, research from Europe suggests the rate of inappropriate procedures is greater than 20% in some settings.[23]

Informed consent Consent with discussion of risks, benefits, and alternatives should be obtained from patients. Patients should be aware of potential risks before undergoing colonoscopy, including bleeding, infection, perforation, sedation adverse events, missed lesions, and intravenous site complications.

Postpolypectomy/postcancer resection surveillance intervals Intervals between surveillance examinations after postpolypectomy and postcancer resection should follow recommended intervals.

Inflammatory bowel disease surveillance intervals Intervals between surveillance examinations in patients with inflammatory bowel disease should follow recommended intervals. Current recommendations on intervals are aimed at achieving optimal balance between risks and benefits for colonoscopy. In the United States, survey data suggest that endoscopists often perform surveillance examinations at intervals that are shorter than those recommended in guidelines.[24] Inappropriate timing for surveillance may occur more often when nongastroenterologists are performing the colonoscopy.[24] In these instances, patients are subject to greater risk for complications with unclear clinical benefit.

Bowel preparation quality All procedure notes should report the quality of the bowel preparation. The quality of a bowel preparation can affect cecal intubation and sensitivity of colonoscopy for neoplastic lesions (both large and small), and lead to repeat examinations.[11,12,25] Poor quality preparations can decrease the effectiveness of colon cancer screening and increase the cost of medical care.[11] Characteristics of the patient population being served may strongly influence the percentage of inadequate bowel preparations.[11] However, the motivation and willingness of an endoscopist to take additional time to suction and avoid the need for a repeat examination may also be a factor. A systematic problem with bowel preparation instructions may lead to suboptimal rates of aborted and repeat procedures.

Intraprocedure
Cecal intubation Reports should document cecal intubation and describe or photodocument cecal landmarks. The extent of the examination should be documented and cecal intubation should occur in 90% or more of all procedures and 95% or more of screening examinations in healthy adults (excluding procedures in which an endoscopist encounters severe colitis, poor preparation quality, severe diverticulosis, or clinical instability).[8,9,26] Although these targets have been shown to be attainable, in some settings only 55% of endoscopists reached the cecum in 90% of cases, and as many as 9% reached the cecum less than 80% of the time.[27]

ADRs Among healthy asymptomatic individuals aged 50 or older who are undergoing screening colonoscopy, an adenoma should be detected in at least 25% of men and at least 15% of women.

More than 60% of colonoscopies in the United States are performed for screening or surveillance of neoplasia.[28] The ADR is considered by the ASGE/ACG Task Force to be the "best neoplasia related indicator" and is one of the most studied quality indicators for colonoscopy.[1,2] Studies have found variation in ADRs in a wide variety of settings.[14,29,30] Colorectal cancers and advanced adenomas are obviously more important clinical outcomes than adenomas, but the ADR has been shown to correlate with the rate of detection of large adenomas, thereby reinforcing its clinical relevance.[14,30] The ADR is perhaps one of the most commonly reported quality measures (albeit typically in academic or research settings), thereby providing substantial data to formulate benchmarks.

Withdrawal times Mean withdrawal time should be 6 minutes or more in patients with intact colons and normal findings.

Rex[31] conducted a study comparing withdrawal time during 10 consecutive procedures by two endoscopists (6 minutes, 41 seconds vs 8 minutes, 55 seconds) with known polyp detection rates, and this study led others to recommend a minimum of 6 minutes. In 2006, Barclay and colleagues[14] found large variation in withdrawal times (3.1–16.8 minutes) among 12 gastroenterologists, and these correlated with variation in adenoma detection. In some settings, however, increasing withdrawal time does not translate into greater polyp yield.[15] Measuring mean withdrawal time may be most appropriate for endoscopists with low rates of adenoma detection as a way to improve performance.

Biopsies for chronic diarrhea Endoscopists should obtain random biopsies in patients with chronic diarrhea. The mucosa of patients with microscopic colitis often appears normal endoscopically. Diagnosing microscopic colitis requires biopsies, and without sampling normal-appearing mucosa, some cases would be missed. The best strategy for obtaining biopsies (with regard to number and distribution) is unclear, but obtaining proximal and distal colon biopsies increases the sensitivity for microscopic colitis.[32]

Biopsy strategy for IBD surveillance Four biopsies should be performed per 10-cm segment of affected colon.

Patients with endoscopic evidence of abnormalities such as scarring develop colon cancer at a higher rate than those without these abnormalities.[33] In patients with IBD, a systematic approach to surveillance biopsies is necessary to optimize the detection of dysplasia. Following the strategy above results in approximately 32 biopsies for panulcerative colitis.

Endoscopic resection of polyps greater than 2 cm Patients with mucosally based pedunculated polyps or sessile polyps smaller than 2 cm should have endoscopic resection attempted or documentation of endoscopic inaccessibility before surgical referral.

In the event of large polyps, endoscopists should attempt to remove polyps endoscopically instead of subjecting patients to surgery. If a difficult polyp is encountered, the endoscopist should obtain adequate photodocumentation and potentially refer the patient to a more experienced endoscopist or a surgeon if the lesion is truly inaccessible.

Postprocedure
Perforation incidence The incidence of perforation should be measured and stratified according to indication.

Perforations are rare during colonoscopy, but approximately 5% of perforations that occur in colonoscopy are fatal.[34] Based on previous studies, a perforation incidence of less than 1 per 500 for all colonoscopies and 1 per 1000 for screening colonoscopies is considered within reason.[35] Although variation in rates of complications, such as perforation and bleeding exists, these indicators should be viewed with some caution. Perforations occur infrequently, and therefore precise estimates for each individual endoscopist may not be reliable. Patient risk factors and procedure complexity should also be taken into account.

Postpolypectomy bleeding Incidence of postpolypectomy bleeding should be measured.

The most common complication of polypectomy is bleeding.[34] Bleeding occurs in fewer than 1% of all cases of polypectomy but in approximately 10% of cases with polyps larger than 2 cm.[34,36] Polyps that are more proximal also have a higher likelihood of bleeding.

Management of postpolypectomy bleeding In the event of continued postpolypectomy bleeding, endoscopic evaluation and management should occur.

When postpolypectomy bleeding occurs, more than 90% of cases can be managed without surgery.[1] Most bleeding will stop spontaneously, but some patients may require a repeat colonoscopy with placement of clips, or injection with cautery.

Reasons for Variation in Quality

Many studies have focused on documenting the existence of variation in colonoscopy quality, but the reasons for this variation have not been clear. Retrospective studies have shown associations between cecal intubation and several factors, including bowel preparation quality, sedation type, colonoscopy setting, and endoscopist factors such as volume and years in practice.[37,38] Others have retrospectively analyzed polyp detection rates and found associations with bowel preparation quality and sedation, among other factors.[38] Some of the variability is certainly due to patient-related factors (eg, demographics, family history) and procedure-related factors (bowel preparation quality, sedation), but a substantial fraction of the variability is also related to endoscopist performance. As a result, quality improvement projects have investigated patient-related changes, organizational arrangements, and endoscopist-related interventions.

Impact of Measurement: Internal Audits and Organizational Changes

In 2004, Ball and colleagues[39] reported one of the first prospective quality improvement projects for colonoscopy. Hoping to improve cecal intubation rates, members of an endoscopy unit in the United Kingdom audited colonoscopy reports over two periods to determine reasons for incomplete examinations. The strategy during the first audit included increasing appointment duration from 20 to 30 minutes, and hospitalization of frail patients for their bowel preparation. This practice led to an increase in cecal intubation rate from 60% to 71.2%. The strategy developed during the second audit included assigning more colonoscopies to the endoscopists with higher cecal intubation rates and having less-successful endoscopists receive further training or stop performing colonoscopies. The group increased their completion rate to 88.1% of all procedures and 93.8% of procedures without a poor bowel preparation, stricture, or obstruction. Not only did the department as a whole improve, but also all of the individual endoscopists who continued to do procedures improved. Although many of the changes were organizational, the authors thought the process of auditing itself also influenced performance.

Imperiali and colleagues[40] used a similar approach to that used by Ball and colleagues,[39] examining a quality improvement project in Italy. They performed six monthly audit cycles from 2001 to 2005. The audits included departmental meetings to discuss standards, review the results of the audit, and develop action plans. Individual endoscopists were informed about their own performance only. One intervention included giving preprocedure sedation instead of on-demand sedation for patients. An approach that differed from the one used by Ball and colleagues[39] was the practice of having more endoscopy sessions for endoscopists with lower performance rates or less experience. The less-skilled endoscopists were also randomly supervised by more-experienced endoscopists, and endoscopists with low polyp detection rates had a personal interview with the head of the unit to discuss the importance of polyps and technical aspects of examination. Additionally if an endoscopist was unable to intubate the cecum, a second endoscopist was instructed to attempt to intubate the cecum, if possible.

Over the study period, the cecal intubation rate increased from 84.6% to 93.1%. The overall polyp detection rate remained about the same, but the range in polyp detection among individual endoscopists decreased. They also acknowledged the possibility that the audit process itself may have been responsible for much of the improvement and reported a slight decrease in cecal intubation during a period when endoscopists were unaware that examinations had been reviewed.

Colonoscopy Technique and Feedback

Harewood and colleagues[41] investigated the issue of feedback on cecal intubation, insertion time, and withdrawal time. On a quarterly basis for almost a year, 58 endoscopists received e-mails communicating their performance and rank compared with their colleagues. The cecal intubation rate increased from 95.3% to 96.2% and insertion time decreased from 10.6 to 9.5 minutes, whereas median withdrawal times did not change significantly. In addition to the e-mails, the group postulated that discussions at divisional meetings may have reinforced the importance of slow withdrawal and careful inspection. They also raised the issue of durability, noting that some of the trends started to reverse toward the end of the study period.

In 2008, Barclay and colleagues[42] investigated a novel quality improvement intervention that involved an emphasis on both withdrawal time and inspection technique. To achieve an 8-minute withdrawal time, they used a digital stopwatch that emitted an audible sound signifying 2-minute increments. To address the issue of inspection technique, the group discussed an article describing techniques (insufflation, suction, inspection of flexures, proximal sides of folds, withdrawal time) and solicited the advice of endoscopists in the group with high ADRs. After the intervention, endoscopists increased the rate of neoplasia detection from 23.5% to 34.7%, which included an approximately 50% increase in the percentage of subjects with at least one adenoma and a 45% increase in the number of advanced adenomas per subject screened. Despite the apparent improvements, the authors found that the endoscopists with the highest ADRs had only intermediate withdrawal times. A retrospective study by other authors failed to identify an increase in polyp detection, using a 7-minute withdrawal protocol.[15]

In one of the largest studies to address the issue of performance improvement, Shaukat and colleagues[43] found that various interventions did not appear to change endoscopists' adenoma detection rates. The authors prospectively collected data on 47,253 screening colonoscopies over 3 years, while instituting five interventions. Interventions included ADR review (blinded and unblinded), education about ADR benchmarks and withdrawal time, discussions between poor performing endoscopists and practice leaders, and financial consequences of not achieving a 6-minute withdrawal time in greater than 95% of colonoscopies.

Although some of the studies above show some improvement, uncertainty still exists regarding the optimal approach to improve endoscopist performance. Elements of inspection thought to impact neoplasia detection include ample insufflation, meticulous evaluation of flexures and proximal sides of folds, adequate suctioning of retained fluid, and withdrawal duration. Recently, operator motivation and fatigue have been suggested as additional factors affecting the yield of colonoscopy. Aside from withdrawal times, most of these features are too ambiguous or difficult to quantify and measure consistently. Furthermore, even if a measure is selected, the optimal frequency and format for feedback is unclear. Finally, if improvements are made, the improvements may not be durable or long-lasting.

High-priority Measures

Although the perfect quality measure does not exist, several measures seem to be particularly useful for improving the quality of colonoscopy: (1) cecal intubation rate, (2) adenoma detection rate, (3) withdrawal time, (4) preparation quality, (5) follow-up recommendations, and (6) ASA classification.

SUMMARY

The emergence of electronic health records and computerized endoscopy report generators should facilitate the use of complete and standardized colonoscopy reports and simplify quality measurement. Pay-for-performance programs and other value-based health care programs have grown dramatically and are expected to continue. Endoscopists have assembled task forces to propose quality indicators and standardized reports and are working on national benchmarking projects, which will allow a better understanding of appropriate thresholds for performance measures. In the future, decisions will need to be made regarding the selection of different sources of measures (health records, billing records, or registries) and issues surrounding access to quality measures. For some, the shift toward standardization and quality measurement will seem to be too great a burden. Others will be hesitant in or fear sharing quality measures with the public or their colleagues. Ultimately, however, as the data regarding the effectiveness of interventions accumulate, it will become apparent that this work benefits patients and the profession.

REFERENCES

1. Rex DK, Petrini JL, Baron TH, et al. Quality indicators for colonoscopy. Gastrointest Endosc 2006;63(Suppl 4):S16–28.
2. Rex DK, Bond JH, Winawer S, et al. Quality in the technical performance of colonoscopy and the continuous quality improvement process for colonoscopy: recommendations of the U.S. Multi-Society Task Force on Colorectal Cancer. Am J Gastroenterol 2002;97(6):1296–308.
3. Lieberman D, Nadel M, Smith RA, et al. Standardized colonoscopy reporting and data system: report of the Quality Assurance Task Group of the National Colorectal Cancer Roundtable. Gastrointest Endosc 2007;65(6):757–66.
4. Mai HD, Sanowski RA, Waring JP. Improved patient care using the A/S/G/E guidelines on quality assurance: a prospective comparative study. Gastrointest Endosc 1991;37(6):597–9.
5. Robertson DJ, Lawrence LB, Shaheen NJ, et al. Quality of colonoscopy reporting: a process of care study. Am J Gastroenterol 2002;97(10):2651–6.
6. Lieberman DA, Faigel DO, Logan JR, et al. Assessment of the quality of colonoscopy reports: results from a multicenter consortium. Gastrointest Endosc 2009; 69(3 Pt 2):645–53.
7. Krist AH, Jones RM, Woolf SH, et al. Timing of repeat colonoscopy: disparity between guidelines and endoscopists' recommendation. Am J Prev Med 2007; 33(6):471–8.
8. Rex DK, Lehman GA, Ulbright TM, et al. Colonic neoplasia in asymptomatic persons with negative fecal occult blood tests: influence of age, gender, and family history. Am J Gastroenterol 1993;88(6):825–31.
9. Lieberman DA, Weiss DG, Bond JH, et al. Use of colonoscopy to screen asymptomatic adults for colorectal cancer. Veterans Affairs Cooperative Study Group 380. N Engl J Med 2000;343(3):162–8.

10. Sharma VK, Nguyen CC, Crowell MD, et al. A national study of cardiopulmonary unplanned events after GI endoscopy. Gastrointest Endosc 2007;66(1):27–34.
11. Rex DK, Imperiale TF, Latinovich DR, et al. Impact of bowel preparation on efficiency and cost of colonoscopy. Am J Gastroenterol 2002;97(7):1696–700.
12. Harewood GC, Sharma VK, de Garmo P. Impact of colonoscopy preparation quality on detection of suspected colonic neoplasia. Gastrointest Endosc 2003; 58(1):76–9.
13. Rabeneck L, Souchek J, El-Serag HB. Survival of colorectal cancer patients hospitalized in the Veterans Affairs Health Care System. Am J Gastroenterol 2003;98(5):1186–92.
14. Barclay RL, Vicari JJ, Doughty AS, et al. Colonoscopic withdrawal times and adenoma detection during screening colonoscopy. N Engl J Med 2006; 355(24):2533–41.
15. Sawhney MS, Cury MS, Neeman N, et al. Effect of institution-wide policy of colonoscopy withdrawal time > or = 7 minutes on polyp detection. Gastroenterology 2008;135(6):1892–8.
16. Wasek S. Are you ahead of the GI QI curve? Available at: www.beckersasc.com. Accessed January 20, 2010.
17. Blumenthal D. Part 1: quality of care–what is it? N Engl J Med 1996;335(12): 891–4.
18. Brook RH, McGlynn EA, Cleary PD. Quality of health care. Part 2: measuring quality of care. N Engl J Med 1996;335(13):966–70.
19. Donabedian A. Explorations in quality assessment and monitoring. The definition of quality and approaches to its assessment, vol. 1. Ann Arbor (MI): Health Administration Press; 1980.
20. Lieberman D. Home repair and colonoscopy: quality counts. Gastrointest Endosc 2006;64(4):563–4.
21. Johanson JF. Quality and outcomes management in gastroenterology. Gastroenterol Clin North Am 1997;26(4):859–71.
22. Johnson DA. Quality Measures Task Force of the American College of, Gastroenterology. Pay for performance: ACG guide for physicians. Am J Gastroenterol 2007;102(10):2119–22.
23. de Bosset V, Froehlich F, Rey JP, et al. Do explicit appropriateness criteria enhance the diagnostic yield of colonoscopy? Endoscopy 2002;34(5):360–8.
24. Mysliwiec PA, Brown ML, Klabunde CN, et al. Are physicians doing too much colonoscopy? A national survey of colorectal surveillance after polypectomy. Ann Intern Med 2004;141(4):264–71.
25. Froehlich F, Wietlisbach V, Gonvers JJ, et al. Impact of colonic cleansing on quality and diagnostic yield of colonoscopy: the European Panel of Appropriateness of Gastrointestinal Endoscopy European multicenter study. Gastrointest Endosc 2005;61(3):378–84.
26. Marshall JB, Barthel JS. The frequency of total colonoscopy and terminal ileal intubation in the 1990s. Gastrointest Endosc 1993;39(4):518–20.
27. Cotton PB, Connor P, McGee D, et al. Colonoscopy: practice variation among 69 hospital-based endoscopists. Gastrointest Endosc 2003;57(3):352–7.
28. Sonnenberg A, Amorosi SL, Lacey MJ, et al. Patterns of endoscopy in the United States: analysis of data from the Centers for Medicare and Medicaid Services and the National Endoscopic Database. Gastrointest Endosc 2008;67(3):489–96.
29. Sanaka MR, Deepinder F, Thota PN, et al. Adenomas are detected more often in morning than in afternoon colonoscopy. Am J Gastroenterol 2009;104(7): 1659–64.

30. Chen SC, Rex DK. Endoscopist can be more powerful than age and male gender in predicting adenoma detection at colonoscopy. Am J Gastroenterol 2007; 102(4):856–61.

31. Rex DK. Colonoscopic withdrawal technique is associated with adenoma miss rates. Gastrointest Endosc 2000;51(1):33–6.

32. Yusoff IF, Ormonde DG, Hoffman NE. Routine colonic mucosal biopsy and ileoscopy increases diagnostic yield in patients undergoing colonoscopy for diarrhea. J Gastroenterol Hepatol 2002;17(3):276–80.

33. Rutter MD, Saunders BP, Wilkinson KH, et al. Cancer surveillance in longstanding ulcerative colitis: endoscopic appearances help predict cancer risk. Gut 2004; 53(12):1813–6.

34. Fruhmorgen P, Demling L. Complications of diagnostic and therapeutic colonoscopy in the Federal Republic of Germany. Results of an inquiry. Endoscopy 1979;11(2):146–50.

35. Gatto NM, Frucht H, Sundararajan V, et al. Risk of perforation after colonoscopy and sigmoidoscopy: a population-based study. J Natl Cancer Inst 2003;95(3): 230–6.

36. Sorbi D, Norton I, Conio M, et al. Postpolypectomy lower GI bleeding: descriptive analysis. Gastrointest Endosc 2000;51(6):690–6.

37. Aslinia F, Uradomo L, Steele A, et al. Quality assessment of colonoscopic cecal intubation: an analysis of 6 years of continuous practice at a university hospital. Am J Gastroenterol 2006;101(4):721–31.

38. Radaelli F, Meucci G, Sgroi G, et al. Italian Association of Hospital Gastroenterologists (AIGO). Am J Gastroenterol 2008;103(5):1122–30.

39. Ball JE, Osbourne J, Jowett S, et al. Quality improvement programme to achieve acceptable colonoscopy completion rates: prospective before and after study. BMJ 2004;329(7467):665–7.

40. Imperiali G, Minoli G, Meucci GM, et al. Effectiveness of a continuous quality improvement program on colonoscopy practice. Endoscopy 2007;39(4):314–8.

41. Harewood GC, Petersen BT, Ott BJ. Prospective assessment of the impact of feedback on colonoscopy performance. Aliment Pharmacol Ther 2006;24(2): 313–8.

42. Barclay RL, Vicari JJ, Greenlaw RL. Effect of a time-dependent colonoscopic withdrawal protocol on adenoma detection during screening colonoscopy. Clin Gastroenterol Hepatol 2008;6(10):1091–8.

43. Shaukat A, Oancea C, Bond JH, et al. Variation in detection of adenomas and polyps by colonoscopy and change over time with a performance improvement program. Clin Gastroenterol Hepatol 2009;7(12):1335–40.

Advanced Systems to Assess Colonoscopy

Piet C. de Groen, MD[a,b]

KEYWORDS

- Colorectal cancer • Colonoscopy • Endoscopist • Quality
- Endoscopic Multimedia Information System

INTRODUCTION: PREVENTION OF COLORECTAL CANCER BY COLONOSCOPY

Colorectal cancer is the second major cause of cancer-related death in the United States.[1] The long time involved in progression of mucosal dysplasia from a small polyp to an invasive cancer, the mucosal shedding of molecules and cells into stool during this process, and the ability to image the colon mucosa using direct inspection or x-ray techniques are features that make early detection and prevention of colorectal cancer possible. Various screening tests, such as digital rectal examination, fecal occult blood testing, double-contrast barium enema, and colonoscopy, have increasingly contributed to the detection of polyps and early cancers. Among these tests, colonoscopy is the most accepted screening method for the detection of colorectal cancer or its precursor lesions and is the only colorectal cancer screening and surveillance technology that allows for diagnostic and therapeutic operations in one procedure. Colonoscopy has contributed to a marked decline in the number of colorectal cancer-related deaths.

THE PROBLEM WITH COLONOSCOPY: NOT ALL COLORECTAL CANCERS ARE PREVENTED

Recent data suggest, however, that there is a significant miss rate for detection of even large polyps and cancers.[2–8] Examples include a double-procedure study from the author's institution where colonoscopy failed to detect 4 out of 5 individual colorectal cancers detected by CT colography,[3] a double-cohort study where colonoscopy detected fewer colorectal cancers than CT colography,[8] a population-based case control study in Canada where colonoscopy did not prevent death from right-sided colorectal cancer,[4] and a screening study from Germany where the repeat

Disclosure: Piet de Groen and Mayo Clinic have a financial interest and hold an equity position in EndoMetric INC, a company that analyzes colonoscopy video streams for features of quality.
[a] Division of Gastroenterology and Hepatology, Department of Internal Medicine, Mayo Clinic College of Medicine, 200 First Street SW, Rochester, MN 55905, USA
[b] Division of Biomedical Statistics and Information, Department of Health Sciences Research, Mayo Clinic College of Medicine, Rochester, MN, USA
E-mail address: pcdegroen@hotmail.com

colonoscopy findings were similar to the case-control study findings in Canada.[6] The conclusion from these and other studies (for a comprehensive summary, see Hewett and colleagues[5]) is that the protective effect of colonoscopy, when used in routine clinical practice, has not lived up to the expectations raised by carefully controlled prospective research studies. Furthermore, the protective effect seems minor or absent for right-sided cancers and at best approximately 70% for left-sided cancers.

ASSUMPTIONS: FACTORS THAT MAY EXPLAIN FAILURES OF COLONOSCOPY

Several factors may contribute to the miss rate. In general, these factors can be divided into those related to the patient, the equipment used, and the endoscopist performing the procedure. A cooperative patient, either due to voluntary control of the patient or due to a moderate amount of sedatives and analgesics, is a requirement for a successful endoscopic examination. Similarly, a colonic anatomy allowing passage of the colonoscope to the cecum is assumed—this is the case in nearly all patients. The patient-related factors that may lower miss rates consist mainly of two important actions: first, discontinuation of any nutrients other than clear liquids for a defined time before the procedure (most often 1–2 days), and, second, strict adherence to a bowel cleansing program 1 to 2 days before the procedure. The desired end result is a colon free of any solid food with either no liquid content or small amounts of highly diluted stool and gastrointestinal juices that are easily aspirated. Although no truly objective measurements for judging colonic preparation exist, a semiquantitive subjective scoring system is used by most endoscopists.[9] The equipment-related protective factors are variable and less dominant than in the past, given the overall quality of the currently available commercial endoscopes. Nevertheless, there are real differences between endoscopes of different manufacturers that can affect the protective effect of colonoscopy. The endoscopist-related protective factors consist mainly of skill set, the inspection time, and the effort exerted to inspect as much of the visible mucosa as possible. At present, skill set is defined as having completed a minimal number of procedures during a formal fellowship; a subset of these procedures should include certain endoscopic diagnostic and therapeutic instrumentations. Formal testing of the acquired skill set does not take place. There is debate about what constitutes optimal inspection time; however, the American Society for Gastroentintestinal Endoscopy (ASGE) and American College of Gastroenterology (ACG) in a consensus document in 2006 suggest that independent of patient, equipment, and endoscopist, at least 6 to 10 minutes should be spent during the withdrawal phase on careful inspection of all visible colon mucosa.[9] The third endoscopist-related factor is the effort to inspect as much of the visible mucosa as possible. Effort is different from skill set. Meticulous effort means that by using all options available, such as torque, lateral (left/right) and vertical (up/down) tip deflexion, aspiration, washing of mucosa, retroflexion, and repeatedly moving through tight angulations, the endoscopist tries to inspect the entire colon mucosa. Current equipment allows inspection of most (>90%–95%) of the colon mucosa (the visible mucosa) during a routine screening colonoscopy in a normal 50-year-old patient if all these techniques are used as required during the procedure. A complete inspection (100% of colon mucosa) is unusual with current endoscopic equipment; inspection of less than 90% to 95% in a well-cleansed colon of a normal 50-year-old patient should lead to questioning the skill set or the level of effort of the endoscopist.

DEFINING QUALITY OF COLONOSCOPY
Metrics that are Being Collected

For each colonoscopic procedure, some data are collected. At the most basic form, data collection consists of a handwritten or dictated free text report with or without a few images in the form of separate photographs. To get paid, a set of billing codes is available, frequently in a separate practice management system. In cases when specimens are obtained, another piece of paper, such as a letter from a pathology laboratory, may hold the final histologic diagnosis. Additional data, in particular data related to quality of the procedure, may not be collected. Meaningful data extraction to examine quality is not possible because this would be prohibitively expensive and provide little or no useful information.

In the most detailed and comprehensive form, detailed electronic data are available with structured information about the indication for the colonoscopy, preprocedure education and instructions, adherence to the bowel preparation regimen, the procedure with all its details, digital images of key anatomic locations and findings, any complications related to the procedure, recovery and discharge, any histologic findings from specimens removed, and suggested follow-up. At present, sophisticated systems allowing all of this are mostly available in large gastroenterology group practices and academic centers. Sometimes practice-, research-, and quality-related data are collected in separate electronic applications; sometimes—and ideally—all these data types are collected in a single application that serves all needs and prevents redundant data collection activity. In reality, in 2010 most endoscopists, whether or not solo practitioners, in a small single specialty group, or in a large multispecialty center, have implemented data collection methods somewhere between basic paper-based and highly comprehensive, digital formats.

Given these descriptions of the wide variety of data collection methods coupled with (1) an absence of any central (ie, federal, state, societal, or insurance) requirements regarding which data should be collected, (2) the voluntary nature of establishing some kind of prospective data collection, (3) the lack of a minimum set of universally agreed-on data types worthy to be collected, (4) the lack of a financial incentive to collect data that would prove quality, and (5) the possible legal ramifications of collecting data that can possibly incriminate the physicians performing the procedures, it is not surprising that most if not all data that currently are collected regarding colonoscopy are simple, limited in quantity, easy to obtain, inexpensive to collect, and not reflecting what actually happened during the procedure.

In 2006, the ASGE and ACG published a consensus report in which these organizations listed a set of minimal criteria related to quality as recommendations.[9] Of these recommendations the following four intraprocedure recommendations are not related to pre-existing disease conditions and best define skill set and effort of the endoscopist during colonoscopy:

1. Cecal intubation rates: visualization of the cecum by notation of landmarks and photo documentation of landmarks should be documented in every procedure.
2. Detection of adenomas in asymptomatic individuals (screening): adenomas should be detected in at least 25% of men and at least 15% women more than 50 years old.
3. Withdrawal times: mean withdrawal time should be at least 6 minutes in colonoscopies with normal results performed in patients with intact colons.
4. Mucosally based pedunculated polyps and sessile polyps less than 2 cm in size should not be sent for surgical resection without an attempt at endoscopic resection or documentation of endoscopic inaccessibility.

The problem with these four recommendations is that they do not reflect the eventual result of colonoscopy—the final state of colon preparation after removal of remaining fecal material, the amount of mucosa inspected, and the completeness of removal of all lesions. If cecal intubation is documented by a good-quality image, then there is solid evidence of the fact that the entire colon was traversed; if an image is not available, the opinion of the endoscopist can be relied on. Finding one or more polyps is not a guarantee that other polyps are not missed. Similarly, spending 6 minutes during withdrawal is not a guarantee that all mucosa was cleaned as needed and inspected. Finally, an attempt at polypectomy of a lesion less than 2 cm is not the same as being able to remove a polyp less than 2 cm without remaining polypoid tissue in (nearly) all cases.

In summary, current intraprocedural quality measures are subjective and do not reflect the effort of the endoscopist to clean, inspect all mucosa, and remove all abnormalities (ie, they do not reflect true quality of colonoscopy). In addition, these limited data provide a false sense of measuring or providing quality and allow easy manipulation (eg, remove one polyp and delay endoscope removal until a withdrawal time of 6 minutes is reached) of data toward an apparently favorable outcome.

Metrics that Should be Collected

Only two things matter when it comes to colonoscopy and colorectal cancer: Was colorectal cancer prevented in the patients who underwent colonoscopy (less morbidity)? and Did the patient live longer due to the intervention (less mortality)? If cancer is prevented but patients do not experience a better quality or longer life, screening is not indicated. Assuming that prevention of colorectal cancer does lead to longer, good quality of life, in my opinion, there are two choices to evaluate colonoscopy (**Fig. 1**). First, when, where, and how colonoscopy fails to prevent colorectal cancer can be measured by calculating the frequency of colorectal cancer despite colonoscopy (CCdC) or the interval colorectal cancer rate. This is not a trivial task—it requires long-term follow-up of a large study population and requires detailed data about the condition of the patient and specimens removed from the patient. Second, whether or not a high-quality colonoscopy was performed can be measured based on evaluation of the entire colonoscopy instead of a limited data set, as is currently the case.

Assessing whether or not colonoscopy prevents colorectal cancer

At the Mayo Clinic, the author and colleagues have created a large database spanning from 1992 to 2009.[10] This database contains all endoscopy, diagnosis, and pathology information about all patients seen at the institution. As data are currently under

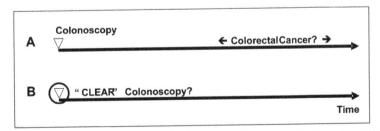

Fig. 1. Options to measure true quality of colonoscopy. The first option is to determine over time whether or not colorectal cancer occurs despite colonoscopy (*A*). The second option is to develop technology that can measure whether or not a high-quality colonoscopy was performed based on the entire colonoscopy (*B*). CLEAR is an acronym for Clean, Look Everywhere and Abnormality Removal, features that define quality of colonoscopy.

review, the results are not disclosed in this article. Several important conclusions, however, are drawn based on the results.

1. First, CCdC is not a random event. Among many factors and features examined, the endoscopist doing the procedure is of key importance because some seem more often involved in CCdC cases than others.
2. Second, most cases of CCdC seem to be truly missed tumors not rapidly growing de novo tumors.
3. Third, these tumors seem to have similar features than tumors that are not missed, suggesting once more that they are truly missed and not rapidly growing de novo tumors.
4. Fourth, withdrawal time duration was not related to number of CCdC, neither was polyp detection rate.
5. Finally, the protective effect for some endoscopists against CCdC extends beyond 3 years and may even extend beyond 5 years, the longest period the author and colleagues have studied thus far.

These preliminary data, from the largest and most detailed study done so far, clearly point to the endoscopist as the key factor determining whether or not a patient develops colorectal cancer in the first 3 to 5 years after a colonoscopy.

Assessing whether or not colonoscopies are of high quality

Measuring failure of prevention of colorectal cancer as the ultimate outcome provides objective, meaningful data but takes many years of careful observation and detailed clinical data acquisition. In addition, patients who underwent a suboptimal colonoscopy may develop and die from colorectal cancer during the observation period, thus not benefiting at all from the quality-control efforts. To address this issue related to colonoscopy, the author and colleagues developed a second approach that uses the entire procedure to determine quality. Instead of taking a few convenient, easily measurable, multiple, procedure-based features, such as cecal intubation rate, adenoma detection rate, and average withdrawal time, the author and colleagues proposed obtaining detailed quality-related information from every colonoscopy representing the entire procedure. Instead of providing an average, subjective, surrogate rating of quality for an endoscopist, which is meaningless for an individual patient, the author and colleagues proposed providing an objective, detailed report of an individual procedure reflecting the actual quality provided to an individual patient.

How is achieving an objective, detailed report for every individual patient proposed? The solution is algorithm-based, automated analysis of the video stream representing the entire procedure. The author and colleagues realize that other important quality features cannot be derived from the video stream, such as preoperative instructions, the amount of discomfort of a patient during the procedure, reasons for not removing polyps, and any follow-up instructions. All of these features are important but become irrelevant in the presence of a poor-quality colonoscopy.

For colonoscopy, one needs to measure from insertion until removal of the endoscope whether or not the endoscopist instituted all efforts reasonably possible to CLEAR the colon of all lesions during the procedure. CLEAR is an acronym that reflects the three important aspects of colonoscopy, which the author and colleagues think define quality:

1. Clean—the patient should adhere to the colon preparation instructions and the endoscopist should remove remaining fecal material. The end result at the time of

withdrawal should be a good or excellent prepared colon as defined in the ASGE and ACG guidelines.
2. *Look Everywhere*—the endoscopist has to actively look behind every fold (working the folds) and move or remove remaining stool to achieve as close to 100% inspection of the colon mucosa.
3. *Abnormality Removal*—the endoscopist has to remove polyps by biopsy forceps, snare polypectomy, or other modalities; lesions left behind may develop into a malignant lesion before a next screening or surveillance procedure is performed.

For each of these three key aspects of colonoscopy, one or more metrics need to be developed to provide a meaningful quality report that truly reflects how well the colonic preparation was after removal of remaining fecal material, how much of the colonic mucosa was well seen, and how completely any premalignant lesions were removed.

ENDOSCOPIC MULTIMEDIA INFORMATION SYSTEM

During the past 7 years, the author and colleagues have developed an automated, innovative system that uses computer-based algorithms to analyze the image stream generated during colonoscopy for specific metrics.[11] This system is named the Endoscopic Multimedia Information System (EMIS). EMIS at present does not interfere with actual colonoscopy because the same image stream analyzed by computer is also displayed on a monitor, allowing a colonoscopist to view the colonic mucosa and perform diagnostic and therapeutic procedures as indicated. The ultimate goal of EMIS, however, is completely automated real-time (ie, during a procedure) analysis of colonoscopy with feedback to the endoscopist to confirm that specific quality milestones have been achieved or to drive endoscopist behavior toward achieving these milestones in case this seems not to happen. EMIS consists of several components, each critical for pursuing the ultimate goal.

EM-Capture

The first component of EMIS is EM-Capture, a set of fully automated, real-time endoscopy video stream capture and file-generation algorithms.[12] The algorithms determine whether or not the image frames are derived from an endoscope with its tip containing the video camera inside the patient. The algorithms use a combination of frame-derived color, movement, and shape aspects in real time to determine absence or presence of an inside-the-patient state. Since May 2007, the author and colleagues have gradually expanded the number of endoscopy rooms equipped with this software from 2 to 13 with outstanding results: under specific conditions, the algorithms remove nearly 100% of all leading outside-the-patient frames and no trailing outside-the-patient frames as programmed. Recording stops after a few continuous minutes of outside-the-patient recording to allow for removal of polyps that are too big to pass via the working channel, change in endoscope, lens cleaning, and so forth. Initially, the author and colleagues recorded a few minutes of the video stream after the endoscope had been removed from the patient to verify that the entire colonocopy procedure has been captured; currently, the author and colleagues record all inside-the-patient images until the time point that the endoscope passes through the anus while verifying that no repeat insertion of the endoscope occurs over the next minutes. In addition, the author and colleagues have verified the number of procedures recorded by the system over a 4-day time span with the number of procedures performed according to endoscopy practice data: comparison showed that the automated, inside-the-patient technology captures every procedure. Comparison showed also that endoscopy practice data—despite best attempts—contained at predictable regularity errors, such as incorrect room assignment and incorrect start and end times of the procedure.

EM-Capture runs on a robotic workstation; this system has no keyboard, mouse, or monitor and is managed remotely by another set of algorithms running on a central server, EM-Central (discussed later). The workstation consists of inexpensive common off-the-shelf hardware: a Core 2 Duo CPU, 4 to 8 GB RAM, two 250-GB or larger hard drives, and a video capture card for total costs, including installation of less than $1500 per endoscopy room. Three cables connect it to (1) 110 V, (2) the image processor of the endoscope, and (3) the intranet. The EM-Capture algorithms run as a component of the operating system; therefore, anyone logging on or off remotely does not interrupt image capture or video file generation. Video file size is variable depending on the length of the procedure. At present, MPEG-2 video files are generated consisting of 30 720 $\times$ 480 pixel color images per second, which results in approximately 1 GB of hard drive space per 20 minutes. Video file capture in high definition format requires substantially more hard drive space per video file.

To summarize, EM-Capture automatically detects when an endoscope enters a patient and provides a collection of video files that represent all endoscopies performed in the rooms where EM-Capture is installed. With EM-Capture, there is a record of every endoscopy from start to finish.

EM-Central

The second component of EMIS is EM-Central, a set of control and scheduling algorithms that reside on a central server.[13] As with EM-Capture on the robotic workstations, EM-Central operates autonomously: it gathers information about the state of the workstations, schedules specific tasks at specific times, and sends e-mails to the programming staff if any of the operating conditions from any of the workstations or the server itself are out of predefined bounds. The EM-Central server also functions as a Web server allowing review of the state of EMIS and access to the various functions of EM-Central via an Internet browser. Currently EM-Central has five main functions:

1. A summary of all captured video files is available under the tab, "Captured Videos." Files can be listed in tabular format or in graphic outline per room and per time period. For instance, a complete overview of a single day, week, month, or year is available per room or for the entire unit (**Fig. 2**).
2. Any automated annotations are shown in the second tab, "Annotated Videos." Drill downs are possible for the annotations and specific images identified (eg, end of insertion, appendix, or instruments) are shown when detected by the algorithms.
3. The state of EMIS hardware and the software programs running on the various workstations and server are shown in the tab, "Machine Status." This allows verification in a single view that all workstations, server, and software are up and running and that enough storage capacity is available.
4. The "Events Log" tab shows a summary of all the actions taken by the central server, such as moving files from capture location to storage server, moving files between workstations, and deleting files.
5. Under "Accounts Management," the manager of the system can set access privileges for people who have access to the system. Depending on role, more or fewer of the system features are available to individual users.

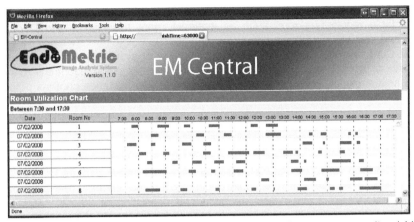

Fig. 2. Screen shot of room use chart for July 2, 2008. Eight endoscopy rooms are listed; blue bars represent the time periods when inside-the-patient events occurred that were detected by EM-Capture and captured and saved as a video files.

EM-Manual

The third component of EMIS is EM-Manual, a manual annotation program.[14] EM-Manual allows extracting single frames or a series of frames as a clip; a clip is a video fragment between by two specific frames (ie, the start and end frames). Using minimal standard terminology (MST), as developed by the European Society of Gastrointestinal Endoscopy, anyone with endoscopic expertise can annotate video files. All MST-based annotations are individual frame based: either the annotation states something about the entire frame (eg, showing a specific anatomic location) or part of a frame is selected using an ellipse and the annotation is limited to that part of the frame (eg, "appendix" in **Fig. 3**).

In addition to MST-based annotations, EM-Manual allows incorporation of custom annotations, used these for two purposes. The first use is to annotate specific features for which algorithms are being developed for machine-based feature recognition. For instance, frames showing the appendiceal orifice are annotated to show the opening of the appendix in the cecum. As MST-based annotations, these are frame-based. The second use is to support specific studies; each study can be supported by one or more study specific tabs. Examples include tabs for overall colon preparation score (according to ASGE and ACG[9]), segmental colon preparation after endoscopic cleansing (Boston bowel preparation scale[15]), key time points (end of insertion, maximal insertion, and end of procedure), and quality of retroflexion (**Fig. 4**). Several of these annotations are video based, some cover the entire video (colon preparation), whereas others may be specific to a small segment (retroflexion).

Annotations are stored in a project folder that resides in the same directory as the video file being annotated. Inside the project folder reside all the annotations, the individual frames that are annotated, and any clips generated from the video file (**Fig. 5**). All annotations are stored in a single extensible markup language (XML) file with extension, APRO (for Arthemis PROject; the original code name of the project[14]). All images are stored in an IMG folder. All clips are stored in a CLIP folder; because a clip is generated from a minimum of two frames, each of which may have annotations, each clip has its own APRO folder with all annotations and images related to the frames inside the clip.

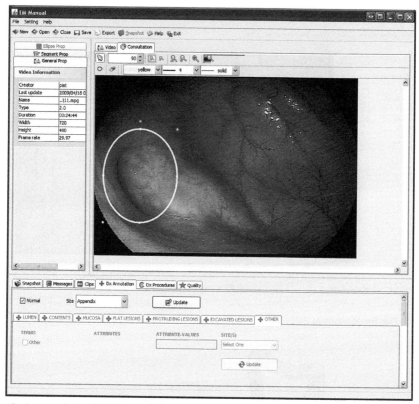

Fig. 3. Screen shot of EM-Manual: frame mode. The left upper frame shows properties of the video, video segments (eg, segmentation based on speech recognition if voice annotation was used during manual video file capture to define colon segments), and annotation tools. The right upper frame shows the consultation panel, allowing annotation of images or components of images. The lower frame shows the various annotation options available. The image component appendix is marked by an ellipse and annotated using MST as "Normal" and Site "Appendix."

All annotations for a series of video files in a single folder can be extracted from the APRO files in the project folders using a dedicated program that generates a single comma-separated values (CSV) file. The CSV file can be loaded into any statistical package for analysis.

EM-Automated

The fourth component of EMIS is EM-Automated, a software package containing algorithms for automatic extraction of endoscopic features.[11] Currently, EM-Automated runs postprocedure (ie, analysis starts after the procedure has been completed). The reason for this is twofold: first, the algorithms take more time than is available during the procedure; and second, the hardware costs to allow real-time annotation until recently were exorbitantly high. Faster algorithms and more powerful workstations at lower cost, however, soon will allow the first algorithms to run in real time. The ultimate goal is to create a real-time version that reliably assesses features related to quality and provides feedback during a colonoscopy.

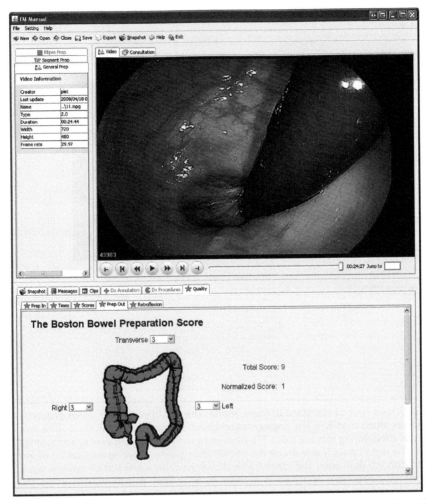

Fig. 4. Screen shot of EM-Manual: video mode. The upper right frame shows the video panel and the lower frame the Boston bowel preparation scale (BBPS) annotation panel. Rapid review of video files is possible in forward and backward play mode. Speed can be increased or decreased in steps of 2 from normal to 32× normal forward speed or 2× normal backward speed using the ">>" and "<<" buttons. Jumping 10 seconds forward or backward is easily achieved using ">|" and "|<" buttons. Jumps to start and end of the video file can be achieved using "|-" and "-|" buttons. Jump to a specific frame can be accomplished by entry of the frame number next to "Jump to." Graphic annotation panels are preferred where possible; in the panel "Prep Out" in the lower frame, a colon model is used for right, transverse, and left colon annotation for BBPS annotation.

To achieve the ultimate goal, EM-Automated needs to complete several steps. First, it needs to determine whether or not the endoscope is inside a patient; currently this is achieved by EM-Capture.[12] Second, it needs to determine whether or not the endoscope is inside a colon; for postprocedure processing, this is irrelevant because the author and colleagues only run the program on video files obtained during colonoscopy. The endoscopy rooms, however, are used for a mix of procedures, including esophagogastroduodenoscopy. For real-time analysis

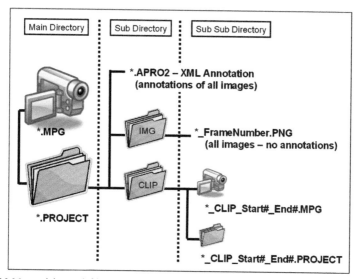

Fig. 5. EM-Manual (APRO) file organization. Video files are stored as *.mpg files. All annotations are stored in a project folder that has the file name of the video file and the file type, "PROJECT." Within the project folder reside the *.APRO2 file (a second more advanced version of an earlier *.APRO format) and subfolders with images selected for annotation and clips generated. A CLIP folder contains the actual clip and the CLIP PROJECT folder; as for the video project folder, the CLIP PROJECT folder contains the clip *.APRO2 file and an image folder. All annotations are contained within the *.APRO2 files and are combined with the video file and images by loading an *.APRO2 file into EM-Manual.

and feedback, the algorithms either need to be instructed that the video stream is from a colonoscopy, or algorithms need to be developed that detect in real time the type of the endoscopy. This work is ongoing. Third, it needs to determine whether or not the images are clear or blurred; analysis of blurred images is unlikely to reveal quality features.[16] Fourth, it needs to determine which part of the clear image consists of colon mucosa and which part consists of remaining fecal material.[17] Finally, it needs to extract several features that are associated with a high-quality colonoscopy and, if these are not present, provide some form of feedback (auditory or visually) to the endoscopist. **Table 1** lists several features for which the author and colleagues have developed algorithms; some run only as postprocedure algorithms, some are already converted to the real-time environment. Some of the preliminary results are discussed.

EMIS RESULTS

The system is still in development; existing algorithms are being optimized, new algorithms are in development, the infrastructure is being altered to allow real-time annotation with feedback, some algorithms are targeted for graphics processing unit (GPU) instead of central processing unit (CPU) processing, and proprietary modules are being replaced by open source modules. The latter two changes are implemented to lower the cost of the hardware and software to make EMIS affordable for every endoscopy unit. Despite that EMIS is far from complete, the author and colleagues already have made several observations.

Table 1
Features for which algorithms have been developed

Feature	Measurement
Image quality	Clear or not clear (blurred)
Stool	Present or absent
Location	Colon segments or unique location
Movement direction	Forward or backward
Speed	Fast or slow
Maximal intubation	Cecum, appendix, terminal ileum, or other
View direction	Forward or lateral
Space-occupying lesion	Present or absent
Instruments	Present or absent
Quadrant coverage histogram	Numeric score
3-D mucosal inspection estimate	Numeric score

Peer Review: EM-Capture Combined with EM-Manual

The author and colleagues have created a huge database of randomly captured as well as specific colonoscopist-derived colonoscopies over the past 5 years using both Fujinon and Olympus equipment. These files are used not only as source for training and test images for algorithm development but also as material for peer review by a varying group of endoscopists. Three preliminary results, currently pending review, can be drawn from analysis of this video file database.

1. There is a large variation in the practice of colonoscopy. In some colonoscopies, endoscopists spend great effort in cleaning remaining fecal material whereas in others most debris is left untouched. In some colonoscopies, endoscopists spend great effort working the folds whereas in others, a single, straight pull backward is observed. Therapeutic maneuvers for similar polypoid lesions can vary from cold biopsy, hot biopsy, cold snare, and hot snare to mucosal resection.
2. There is consensus among endoscopists as assessed by peer review regarding important aspects of quality. Preliminary peer review data show that endoscopists agree strongly when a colonoscopy is performed with high quality.[18] Agreement among endoscopists is less marked when certain features of quality are present but others not (eg, excellent fecal material removal without working the folds or inspecting angulations). This likely reflects a difference of endoscopists' expectations, in other words, a difference in individual definition of what defines high quality.
3. Some endoscopists are significantly and persistently better in performing high-quality colonoscopy examinations than others. Again, these data are under review, but the conclusion is obvious: endoscopists are not all equal.

These preliminary results strongly support the author and colleagues' conviction: an objective review and feedback process—ideally during the examination—is needed of every colonoscopy to guarantee that every patient undergoes an examination that includes a minimal set of quality deliverables.

Computer-Based Review: EM-Capture Combined with EM-Automated

In fall of 2010, the author and colleagues will start rollout at the Mayo Clinic of a system that performs completely automated video stream capture and postprocedure analysis. The system consists of EM-Capture, EM-Central, and a postprocedure version of EM-Automated. EM-Central will monitor EM-Capture and, when EM-Capture is done for the day, direct EM-Automated to execute several algorithms that will derive metrics regarding the following aspects of colonoscopy:

- Image quality—fraction of images that are clear in each specific phase of the procedure
- Mucosal preparation—fraction of clear images with stool and within images with stool the fraction of the image that shows stool (**Fig. 6**)
- Maximal extent—time point when insertion phase ends and withdrawal phase starts
- Appendix—time points and images when appendix is detected
- Back and forth movements—the number of times the endoscope changes direction in forward-backward direction
- Quadrant coverage histogram[19]—a score that consists of the number of times the endoscope tip traverses all quadrants of the colon for a predefined lateral deflection from the central axis; this score is the author and colleagues' first effort at measuring working the folds (**Fig. 7**).

For each of these metrics, the author and colleagues have developed, tested, and implemented computer-based algorithms. In each case, the same method was followed: a set of video files or images was created that contained the features for which algorithms were being created. These were divided in training and test bed. The training files or images were used to develop and train the algorithms; the test bed was used to determine the sensitivity and specificity of the mature algorithms. The author and colleagues created algorithms for an extensive list of features, not all of which will be implemented in the first rollout of EM-Capture combined with EM-Manual (see **Table 1**).

Each of these metrics can be studied per time or anatomic—if known—segment, providing far more accurate, objective information about the procedure than any other method. A copy of several images (eg, one clear image every 15 seconds) and images of key events, such as maximal extent and appendix, can automatically be stored to provide a succinct summary of the procedure without taking up much disk space. In addition, gaming the system, easily achieved under current guidelines (eg, watching the clock for 6 minutes during withdrawal), will be difficult if not impossible. Saving the entire video file, if only for 2 to 4 weeks, to allow review by health care providers

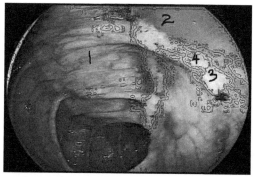

Fig. 6. Example of automated stool detection. Region 1 is clear mucosa; regions 2, 3, and 4 are mucosa covered with stool.

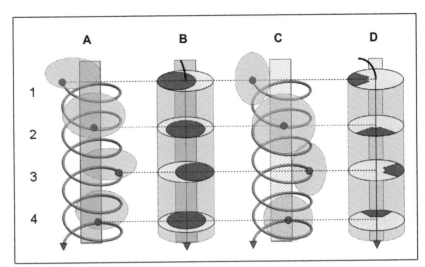

Fig. 7. Quadrant coverage histogram: Circumferential withdrawal: A and C show the spiral shape of the movement of the tip of the endoscope. B and D show the visual field in red. A and B reflect views in which the distant proximal colon is visible; C and D reflect views in which the distant proximal colon is absent and only colon wall is seen. Position 1 shows a left lateral quadrant view, position 2 a superior quadrant view, position 3 a right lateral quadrant view, and position 4 an inferior quadrant view; endoscopic views are from bottom to top of figure. The green bars in A and B indicate the distant proximal colon visible in all positions; hatched green bars in C and D indicate the distant proximal colon that is not visible in any position. The quadrant coverage histogram algorithm counts the number of times the tip of the endoscope passes through all four quadrants at a specific deflexion from the center. (*From* Liu D, Cao Y, Tavanapong W, et al. Quadrant coverage histogram: a new method for measuring quality of colonoscopic procedures. Conf Proc IEEE Eng Med Biol Soc 2007;1:3470-3; with permission.)

or patients is likely to encourage high-quality examinations because nobody wishes to create a semipermanent record of a low-quality colonoscopy.

Whatever the final implementation of the EMIS technology, future studies will need to investigate whether or not (1) EMIS can measure differences in quality of colonoscopy and (2) whether or not a high score from EMIS means that a high-quality colonoscopy was done. The EM-Manual derived scores will be compared with the EM-Automated derived scores in formal, blinded research studies.

Computer-Based Feedback: EM-Capture and Real-Time EM-Automated

In 2012, the author and colleagues plan to roll out a system that does image capture, quality analysis, and polyp detection in real time. This requires three major advances. First, a new computer infrastructure needs to be created that permits advanced, complex real-time image analysis at an affordable price. Such an infrastructure does not yet exist. However, tremendous advances in hardware and software—multiprocessor CPU chips, multithreading 64-bit operating systems, multiprocessor GPU chips, and new software to effectively and easily use these massively multithreaded manycore GPU chips—are occurring while at the same time costs are rapidly decreasing. Second, a fast polyp detection technique needs to be developed. The author and colleagues, as well as others, have developed several polyp detection techniques, some based on shape, some based on texture. None of these techniques, however, are either fast enough or of high enough accuracy to allow real-time detection when using low-cost capture stations. Affordable, multiprocessor CPU/GPU systems will allow implementing polyp detection techniques in real time. Third, a timely and easily understood real-time feedback method needs to be developed. Feedback needs to be provided as soon as possible when a persistent deviation from predefined guidelines occurs. Alternatively, feedback should not detract and interfere with normal workflow. The author and colleagues are working on two types of feedback: visual, by providing overlay projection on the monitor visible to all in the endoscopy room, and auditory, by providing a voice message via earphone for private, endoscopist-only feedback. Finally, the message should be simple and clear, and the endoscopist should be able to respond to the message with a predictable endoscopic action that is considered to improve quality and can be measured using EMIS technology. **Fig. 8** provides a schematic view of the real-time solution. A first effort at real-time feedback will occur in 2010: the author and colleagues are planning to provide real-time feedback related to the fact that retroflexion in the rectum has been performed and, if this is the case, whether or not the images show clear images of the entire mucosa surrounding the endoscope coming through the anal canal.

FUTURE PLANS

Preliminary data from manual review of colonoscopy video files show that most endo-scopists try to remove most polyps that are detected and visualized. Not all polyps seem to be removed and not all polyps are completely removed, but there may be reasons for leaving behind polyps (eg, patient to have surgery, patient on anticoagula-tion, and so forth) or part of polyps (eg, patient becomes hemodynamically unstable and procedure is aborted) that are not obvious from only analyzing the video stream. All endoscopists who have shown interest in the author and colleagues' system seem to agree on one feature they wished were available: a metric that shows how much of the colon mucosa actually was inspected. To estimate this, the author and colleagues have developed a new method that generates a 3-D image out of 2-D images.[20] That

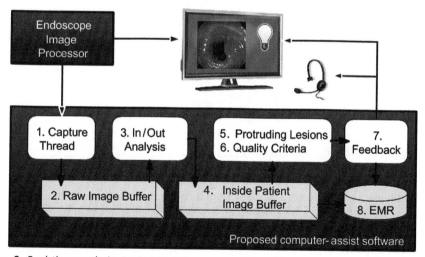

Fig. 8. Real-time analysis. During real-time analysis, the video stream is analyzed first for inside/outside patient state. If the endoscope is inside a patient, the images are kept in the buffer and analyzed for protruding lesions and quality criteria. Feedback is provided either visually or auditory; the feedback and the response to the feedback are stored and can be imported into the electronic medical record (EMR) if desired.

which cannot be seen cannot be measured accurately, but by using a surface interpolation technique and several logical assumptions, the author and colleagues think that those areas of the colon that may have escaped inspection can be estimated with surprising usefulness and clarity. The colon is able to be displayed in 3-D similar to CT colography and then virtual inspection—fly through—allowed of the simulated colon with an estimate of mucosa visualized as well as not visualized given a specific endoscope lens and presence or absence of tip deflection (ie, simulating the effort to look behind folds [**Fig. 9**]). The goal is to make this technique available in real-time providing periodic feedback (eg, once every several minutes or once every colon segment) to the endoscopist and thus provide the endoscopist the opportunity to go back and inspect areas previously missed.

The ultimate goal of the author and colleagues' work is to develop an automated, real-time, video stream–based analysis system that provides feedback to the endoscopist as needed to guarantee that each endoscopic procedure is of high quality. The system should be transparent for those who perform a high-quality procedure and provide suggestions to those who are not meeting established, scientifically verified minimal criteria. By off-loading repetitive, calculation-intensive algorithms to coprocessors on common off-the-shelf graphic cards and using—where possible—open source software components, the author and colleagues plan to keep the

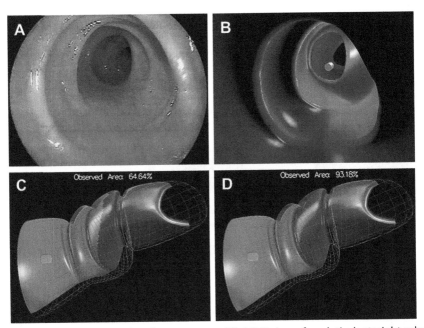

Fig. 9. Estimation of mucosal surface area seen. (*A*) A 2-D view of a relatively straight colon. (*B*) A 3-D representation in 2-D of (*A*). (*C*) A 3-D representation of (*A*) before fly through of the tip of the endoscope (*gray/white cylinder*). (*D*) A 3-D representation of (*A*) after fly through. Pink areas represent mucosa that can be inspected before fly through (*C*) and has been inspected after fly through (*D*) without tip deflection. Green areas represent mucosa that has not been inspected. The simulation estimates that in a relatively straight colon approximately 93% of the mucosal surface can be inspected with fly through without lateral tip deflection (*D*). (*From* Hong D, Tavanapong W, Wong J, et al. 3D Reconstruction of colon segments from colonoscopy images. In: IEEE Int'l Conf on Bioinformatics and Bioengineering. Taiwan 2009; p. 53-60.)

system affordable. All data, including any feedback provided and the response of the endoscopist to the feedback, will be recorded and can be—if desired—stored as part of a permanent electronic medical record.

The author and colleagues need to prove that such a system decreases the incidence of CCdC, provides all patients with a high-quality colonoscopy, and hopefully turns suboptimal endoscopists into good or excellent colonoscopists. An additional beneficial side effect of the technology likely will be that the interval between colonoscopies can be extended due to more effective and complete clearing of the colon, thereby reducing costs. Therefore, all parties involved—the patient, the endoscopist and the payers—in the long run stand to benefit from the system.

SUMMARY

In summary, the protective effect of colonoscopy is dependent on patient-, equipment-, and endoscopist-related factors. Of these three factors, endoscopist- and patient-related factors show most variation and are most difficult to assess. At present, objective methods to assess adequacy of the colonic preparation, the acquired skill set of the endoscopist (either at the end of training or after several years in practice), the true inspection time during withdrawal, and the effort exerted by the endoscopist to inspect all visible mucosa do not exist.

The author and colleagues present two methods to measure a more accurate estimation of quality of colonoscopy. The first method is to study the long-term outcome of all patients for a specific endoscopist; the measurement is CCdG, and the goal for the endoscopist is to detect and treat all precursor lesions and, therefore, to have no patients with CCdG. Because this method relies on long-term follow-up and does not provide protection for patients of endoscopists who perform less than optimal quality colonoscopy, the author and colleagues have developed a second method that automatically assesses a combination of intraprocedural factors that are commonly thought to greatly influence overall quality and outcome of a colonoscopic procedure. This second method currently is postprocedure, but the author and colleagues are converting it to real time (ie, during the procedure) with feedback to the endoscopist as needed. Finally, a combination of these two methods, as part of a rigorous prospective study, is required to validate that real-time analysis and feedback protects patients in the long term from CCdC.

ACKNOWLEDGMENTS

This review discusses some research results that have been submitted for publication. I am indebted to Rohit Gupta and Vipin Kumar from the University of Minnesota in Minneapolis, Minnesota; Monique van Leerdam from the Erasmus University in Rotterdam, The Netherlands; Wallapak Tavanapong and Johnny Wong from Iowa State University in Ames, Iowa; JungHwan Oh from the University of North Texas in Denton, Texas; and Johan Bakken and Felicity Enders from the Mayo Clinic in Rochester, Minnesota; for their contributions. This work was supported by grants from the National Science Foundation, the Agency for Healthcare Research and Quality, the National Institute of Diabetes and Digestive and Kidney Diseases, and the Mayo Clinic.

REFERENCES

1. Jemal A, Siegel R, Ward E, et al. Cancer statistics, 2009. CA Cancer J Clin 2009; 59(4):225–49.

2. Bressler B, Paszat LF, Chen Z, et al. Rates of new or missed colorectal cancers after colonoscopy and their risk factors: a population-based analysis. Gastroenterology 2007;132(1):96–102.

3. Johnson CD, Fletcher JG, MacCarty RL, et al. Effect of slice thickness and primary 2D versus 3D virtual dissection on colorectal lesion detection at CT colonography in 452 asymptomatic adults. AJR Am J Roentgenol 2007;189(3): 672–80.

4. Baxter NN, Goldwasser MA, Paszat LF, et al. Association of colonoscopy and death from colorectal cancer. Ann Intern Med 2009;150(1):1.

5. Hewett DG, Kahi CJ, Rex DK. Does colonoscopy work? J Natl Compr Canc Netw 2010;8(1):67–77.

6. Brenner H, Hoffmeister M, Arndt V, et al. Protection from right- and left-sided colorectal neoplasms after colonoscopy: population-based study. J Natl Cancer Inst 2010;102(2):89–95.

7. Singh H, Nugent Z, Mahmud SM, et al. Predictors of colorectal cancer after negative colonoscopy: a population-based study. Am J Gastroenterol 2010;105(3): 663–73 [quiz: 74].

8. Kim DH, Pickhardt PJ, Taylor AJ, et al. CT colonography versus colonoscopy for the detection of advanced neoplasia. N Engl J Med 2007;357(14):1403–12.

9. Rex DK, Petrini JL, Baron TH, et al. Quality indicators for colonoscopy. Gastrointest Endosc 2006;63(Suppl 4):S16–28.

10. Gupta R, Steinbach M, Ballman KV, et al. Colorectal cancer despite colonoscopy: critical is the endoscopist, not the withdrawal time. Gastroenterology 2009;136(5 Suppl 1):A-55.

11. Oh J, Hwang S, Cao Y, et al. Measuring objective quality of colonoscopy. IEEE Trans Biomed Eng 2009;56(9):2190–6.

12. Stanek SR, Tavanapong W, Wong JS, et al. Automatic real-time capture and segmentation of endoscopy video. Proc SPIE 2008;6919:69190X.

13. Zhang M, Wong J, Tavanapong W, et al. Deadline-constrained media uploading systems. Multimed Tool Appl 2007;38:51–74.

14. Liu D, Cao Y, Kim KH, et al. Arthemis: annotation software in an integrated capturing and analysis system for colonoscopy. Comput Methods Programs Biomed 2007;88(2):152–63.

15. Lai EJ, Calderwood AH, Doros G, et al. The Boston bowel preparation scale: a valid and reliable instrument for colonoscopy-oriented research. Gastrointest Endosc 2009;69(3 Pt 2):620–5.

16. Oh J, Hwang S, Lee J, et al. Informative frame classification for endoscopy video. Med Image Anal 2007;11(2):110–27.

17. Hwang S, Oh J, Tavanapong W, et al. Stool detection in colonoscopy videos. In: Principe JC, Ostrom HV, editors. International Conference of the IEEE Engineering in Medicine and Biology Society. Vancouver (Canada), 2008. p. 3004–7.

18. Bakken J, van Leerdam M, Enders F, et al. Colonoscopy peer review utilizing automated video capture. Am J Gastroenterol 2009;104(Suppl 3):s522.

19. Liu D, Cao Y, Tavanapong W, et al. Quadrant coverage histogram: a new method for measuring quality of colonoscopic procedures. Conf Proc IEEE Eng Med Biol Soc 2007;1:3470–3.

20. Hong D, Tavanapong W, Wong J, et al. 3D Reconstruction of colon segments from colonoscopy images. In: Tsai JJP, Sheu PCY, Hsiao HCW, editors. IEEE International Conference on Bioinformatics and Bioengineering. IEEE Computer Society; 2009. Taichung (Taiwan), June 22–24, 2009. p. 53–60.

The Use of Databases and Registries to Enhance Colonoscopy Quality

Judith R. Logan, MD[a],*, David A. Lieberman, MD[b]

KEYWORDS

- Clinical registries • Administrative databases
- Electronic health record

Studies that help define quality and population-based quality measurement both require large sources of data, including administrative databases, population-based surveys, disease or procedure-specific registries, and data aggregated from electronic health records. It is evident to all attempting to write evidence-based quality measures that ongoing studies are needed to define quality. Population-based quality measurement can enhance quality through promoting system change. Measurement of group or individual provider quality, although not producing quality by the measurement process alone, can enhance quality by motivating the providers to change behavior. As with population-based studies, measurement of individual quality often requires use of administrative data, quality-oriented registries, or electronic health records as data sources. The purpose of this article is to explore the use of these data sources to enhance quality, look for current examples of their use, and then consider the advantages and challenges of each.

Administrative databases, registries, and clinical databases are defined and differentiated by an axis representing purpose, administrative databases primarily used for billing, health care system enrollment and management, clinical databases as record repositories and for communication of clinical care, and registries as limited collections of data for specific research purposes. But there is significant overlap, truly a spectrum of large datasets available for enhancing quality; registries may contain data that is considered administrative, such as billing codes, along with data extracted from electronic health records, and so forth. For purposes of this article, the authors consider administrative data to be any data, coded or otherwise,

The authors have nothing to disclose.
[a] Department of Medical Informatics and Clinical Epidemiology, Oregon Health & Science University, Mailcode: BICC, 3181 SW Sam Jackson Park Road, Portland, OR 97239, USA
[b] Division of Gastroenterology and Hepatology, Department of Medicine, Oregon Health & Science University, Mailcode: L461, 3181 SW Sam Jackson Park Road, Portland, OR 97239, USA
* Corresponding author.
E-mail address: loganju@ohsu.edu

Gastrointest Endoscopy Clin N Am 20 (2010) 717–734
doi:10.1016/j.giec.2010.07.007
1052-5157/10/$ – see front matter © 2010 Elsevier Inc. All rights reserved.

collected for purposes of billing, scheduling, ordering services or supplies, or for compliance with regulatory agencies. They contain demographics and plausible records of medications dispensed and immunizations given. Registries are created for research, but differ from protocol-driven research databases by intent, used primarily for observational rather than interventional research. Although research using registries is still driven by research hypotheses,[1] by nature they can be used to answer multiple questions and may evolve over time. Although registries usually include data that is also contained in the clinical record, registry data is often categorical and more analytically structured than the same data as captured during clinical care. Clinical databases are created to support clinical care, and although discrete (and therefore computable) data is the rule for laboratory results[2–4] and demographics, narrative text is the rule for most documentation, including that of clinical encounters, pathology, and radiology reports and even of clinical orders, such as for pharmaceuticals.

Data gathered for all 3 purposes, however, can be used to enhance quality along a second axis representing the types of quality enhancement. *Discovery of quality* or lack of quality in the population can result in hypotheses for appropriate quality measures. *Measuring disparities* in quality in the population can promote measures for improving population health. *Quantifying quality* within health care facilities or plans, by provider group or individual provider, can promote quality through feedback, pay for performance, or requirements for licensing and certification.

THE USE OF LARGE DATABASES TO ENHANCE QUALITY: THE NATIONAL HEALTHCARE QUALITY REPORT EXAMPLE

Large databases result from data collected for administrative purposes, from surveys performed for developing national agendas and other reasons, or from disease or procedure-specific registries. The authors are familiar with the use of these large databases for epidemiologic studies,[5] including studies of the burden of gastrointestinal disease.[6–9] The National Healthcare Quality Reports (NHQR) are an example of use of these sources for discovery of quality and of the trends in quality care.

The NHQRs have resulted from a 1999 congressional mandate to the Agency for Healthcare Research and Quality (AHRQ) and have been developed in coordination with the Department of Health and Human Services. The most recent report available containing measures for colorectal cancer screening is the 2008 report,[10] which includes data from 2005 with comparison data from as early as 1999, depending upon the measure. The 2008 NHQR used 33 databases (**Box 1**) to report on process and outcome measures aggregated at the national and state level. As defined in this report, process measures "track the receipt of medical services"; whereas, outcome measures "in part reflect the results of medical care."[10] Of 40 core report measures and 9 composite measures, 3 core measures for colorectal cancer are reported every other year along with a fourth noncore measure endorsed by the National Quality Forum[11] concerning surgical resection of colorectal cancer. The 2008 report measures and findings include the following information:

- Colorectal cancer screening: adults aged 50 years and older who ever received colorectal cancer screening (colonoscopy, sigmoidoscopy, proctoscopy, or fecal occult blood test)
    - In 2005, 55.5% of adults aged 50 years and older (49.2% in individuals aged 50–64 years, 63.1% for adults aged 65 years and older) had received screening for colorectal cancer. This result was an increase from 49.8% in 2000.

- Advanced stage colorectal cancer: colorectal cancer diagnosed at advance stage (tumors diagnosed at regional or distant site) per 100,000 population aged 50 years and older

  In 2005, 80.8 advanced stage colorectal tumors were diagnosed per 100,000 population. There has been a steady decrease in this number since first reported in 2000 at 95.2 per 100,000 population.

- Colorectal cancer mortality: colorectal cancer deaths per 100,000 population per year

  The United States Healthy People 2010 goal for colorectal cancer deaths is 13.7 per 100,000. A steady downward trend has occurred since 1999 with 17.5 per 100,000 in 2005.

The application of large databases for quality enhancement requires significant resources and analytical expertise. The quality of these data sources must be judged in the same ways as all data found in clinical and research settings, and accurate interpretation of the data demands availability of analysts with appropriate expertise with both the sources' database structure and content. The possible effects of such reporting, however, can be seen in system changes after feedback of measurement results to providers; national, state, and local administrative units and health care organizations; and from the informed implementation of clinical decision support systems that support just-in-time quality care.[12]

CHALLENGES IN THE USE OF ADMINISTRATIVE DATA

The credibility of administrative data, which is usually insurance claims data, for quality reporting and research has long been the subject of debate.[13–16] The term *powerful* is often used to describe the role of administrative data in studying population-based patterns of health, disease, and medical care.[13] This powerful data has potential advantages for research and quality, including the ability to measure large samples of geographically dispersed patients, the ability to assemble longitudinal records of both inpatient and outpatient care and across providers, and the fact that the data is already collected and inexpensive for investigators to obtain relative to the collection of clinical data through chart abstraction.[17]

Administrative data, however, is not collected for the purpose of measuring quality and its validity for this purpose has been questioned. Of particular concern with US administrative databases is the use of 2 coding systems: the International Classification of Diseases, 9th Revision, Clinical Modification (ICD-9-CM), which is used for coding diagnoses by both hospitals and physicians and for coding procedures by hospitals; and the American Medical Association's Current Procedural Terminology (CPT), which is used by physicians for coding procedures. For insightful review of the use of administrative data for assessing quality across a decade, see the review and editorial by Iezzoni.[14,15] This author describes how administrative files often explicitly aim to minimize data collection by limiting the number of slots available for codes that may affect completeness of comorbidity documentation, and that coding inaccuracy may occur in an effort to maximize payment, as from the Medicare Prospective Payment System using diagnosis-related groups, or to minimize the perception of poor quality through underreporting of complications. The coding systems for procedures (ICD-9-CM for hospitals and CPT for physicians) do not readily link, "hindering comparisons between hospital-generated and physician-generated data."[14] Until 2007, diagnoses present on admission could not be differentiated from complications occurring during hospitalization in Medicare billing data.

Box 1
Databases used in the 2008 National Healthcare Quality Report

Survey data collected from populations

- AHRQ, Medical Expenditure Panel Survey, 2000 to 2005
- US Centers for Disease Control and Prevention (CDC), Behavioral Risk Factor Surveillance System, 2001 to 2006
- CDC-National Center for Health Statistics (NCHS), National Health and Nutrition Examination Survey, 1999 to 2006
- CDC-NCHS, National Health Interview Survey, 1998 to 2006
- CDC-NCHS/National Immunization Program, National Immunization Survey, 1998 to 2006
- Centers for Medicare and Medicaid Services (CMS), Medicare Current Beneficiary Survey, 1998 to 2004
- National Center for Education Statistics, National Assessment of Adult Literacy, Health Literacy Component, 2003
- National Hospice and Palliative Care Organization, Family Evaluation of Hospice Care, 2005 to 2007
- National Institutes of Health (NIH), National Institute of Mental Health, Collaborative Psychiatric Epidemiology Surveys, 2001 to 2003
- Substance Abuse and Mental Health Services Administration, National Survey on Drug Use and Health, 2002 to 2006
- US Census Bureau, American Community Survey, 2006

Data collected from samples of health care facilities and providers

- American Cancer Society and American College of Surgeons, National Cancer database, 1999 to 2005
- CDC-NCHS, National Ambulatory Medical Care Survey, 1997–2006
- CDC-NCHS, National Hospital Ambulatory Medical Care Survey-Emergency Department, 1997 to 2006
- CDC-NCHS, National Hospital Ambulatory Medical Care Survey-Outpatient Department, 1997 to 2006
- CDC-NCHS, National Hospital Discharge Survey, 1998 to 2006
- CMS, End Stage Renal Disease Clinical Performance Measures Project, 2001 to 2006

Data extracted from data systems of health care organizations

- AHRQ, Healthcare Cost and Use Project, Nationwide Inpatient Sample, 1994, 1997, 2000 to 2005, and State Inpatient Databases, 2001 to 2005
- CMS, Home Health Outcomes and Assessment Information Set, 2002 to 2006
- CMS, Hospital Compare, 2006
- CMS, Medicare Patient Safety Monitoring System, 2004 to 2006
- CMS, Nursing Home Minimum Data Set, 1999 to 2006
- CMS, Quality Improvement Organization program, Hospital Quality Alliance measures, 2002 to 2006
- HIV Research Network data, 2003 to 2005
- Indian Health Service, National Patient Information Reporting System, 2002 to 2005
- National Committee for Quality Assurance, Health Plan Employer Data and Information Set, 2001 to 2005

- NIH, United States Renal Data System, 1998–2004

- SAMHSA, Treatment Episode Data Set, 2002–2005

Data from surveillance and vital statistics systems

- CDC-National Center for HIV, Viral Hepatitis, STD, and TB Prevention, HIV/AIDS Reporting System, 1998 to 2006

- CDC-National Center for HIV, STD, and TB Prevention, TB Surveillance System, 1999 to 2004

- CDC-National Program of Cancer Registries, 2000 to 2004

- CDC-NCHS, National Vital Statistics System, 1999 to 2005

- NIH-National Cancer Institute, Surveillance, Epidemiology, and End Results program, 2000 to 2005

Data from National Healthcare Quality Report 2008. Agency for Healthcare Research and Quality. Available at: http://www.ahrq.gov/qual/nhqr08/nhqr08.pdf. Accessed February 14, 2010.

Administrative data has been shown in some circumstances to lack either specificity or sensitivity for identifying conditions important in quality measurement. Jollis and colleagues[17] demonstrated that claims data failed to identify more than 50% of patients with any of several important conditions when compared with a clinical information system. Other studies reported by Jollis found that clinical criteria for acute myocardial infarction were found in only 43% to 87% of records having this diagnosis coded at discharge. Keating and colleagues[18] used 3 accepted measures of quality care for diabetes and compared the use of administrative data alone with administrative data plus medical record data from 3 health plans. Underdetection of quality indicators was noted for all 3 health systems using administrative data alone, and, importantly, the ranking of the health systems changed for some indicators when data from both sources was used. In addition, the degree of underdetection varied by patient age and race, pointing out the complexity of accurate quality reporting.

In quality measurement, inclusion of cases in the denominator of a measure that do not accurately represent the condition being tested can falsely conclude underperformance on the measure. Solberg and colleagues[19] explored algorithms for improving the positive predictive value of case identification for 3 conditions using administrative records, after discovering that using a single code to identify cases of diabetes might include up to 80% of cases without diabetes. The algorithms developed for accurate case identification required for all conditions that more than a single code be used. For example, accurately identifying cases with diabetes required either 2 or more outpatient or 1 inpatient ICD-9 code for diabetes in a year or a filled prescription for a diabetes-specific medication (excluding a medication that may be used for diabetes and other conditions), and assumed health plan enrollment for at least 11 months of the year being studied.

Incomplete physician documentation can lead to omissions in administrative codes. Davenport and colleagues[20] compared data on surgeries performed at a single institution as recorded in 2 volunteer systems; the University HealthSystem Consortium Clinical Database,[21] which relies on administrative data, primarily ICD-9 codes entered by hospital billing coders; and the National Surgical Quality Improvement Program,[22] which requires that nurses extract the data from the medical record and code it to risk and outcome variables specifically designed for risk-adjusting surgical outcomes. To justify billing, the billing coders are required to code only conditions and procedures that are clearly documented by physicians, sometimes with specific wording, and therefore cannot use conditions and procedures that are identifiable in nursing and other notes.

Ultimately, the lesson learned is that for administrative data to be used for enhancing quality, its use is subject to the same caveats as for successful conduct of research using any large databases; the investigator must have adequate knowledge of the database structure and its contents, in particular, knowledge of the completeness and accuracy of the data contained and must be cautious in the conclusions drawn. Comparison with clinical databases, including chart validation of a subset of cases of interest, should be considered before determining the accuracy of the codes used,[5,16] although this may be untenable for many administrative databases, especially those in the public domain without the ability to link to identified health records.

A recent study on the association of colonoscopy and death from colorectal cancer (CRC)[23] highlights some of the advantages and limitations of using administrative databases in research. The design was a population-based case-control study in Ontario, using administrative claims to ascertain exposure to colonoscopy and diagnosis of CRC. Exposures in more than 10,000 case subjects (with CRC) were compared with controls matched for age, sex, geographic region, and socio-economic status. The analysis found that subjects with prior colonoscopy had a 67% reduction in risk of death from left-sided CRC compared with controls and no reduction in risk of death from right-sided cancer. The study raised serious concerns about the potential benefits of screening with colonoscopy.

The strengths of this study include the large number of cases with matched controls. Cases and controls came from typical practice settings, suggesting that data could be generalizable. There is some biologic plausibility to the outcome; cancers of the right colon may be biologically different from distal cancers.

The limitations are also significant and are related to the administrative nature of the data. First, the indications for colonoscopy are unknown. It is unlikely that most examinations were screening examinations during the time period of the study (1992–2003), when little screening colonoscopy was performed in Canada. If rectal bleeding was a common indication, the procedures may have been more likely to detect left-sided lesions because these may present with bleeding, and exerted a more protective effect in the left colon because of selection bias. A second limitation is that we cannot determine the quality or completeness of the colonoscopy examination from the administrative database. For example, it is quite possible that some examinations coded as colonoscopy were incomplete, and did not fully visualize the proximal colon. It is also possible that the bowel prep was poor in the proximal colon. In both situations, the outcome could be a poor quality examination of the proximal colon, which could result in failure of colonoscopy to exert a protective effect. Finally, it is not known if there were polyps seen but not removed at colonoscopy. Based on the National Polyp Study,[24] polypectomy was associated with a lower than expected rate of CRC during surveillance, suggesting that one of the primary benefits of colonoscopy is the detection and removal of cancer precursor lesions. Using this administrative database, the authors cannot determine if all detected polyps were removed. The limitations of this study are largely caused by the lack of data precision in the administrative database, and potentially compromise the outcome. The authors cannot determine if the result is caused by poor quality colonoscopy, or true biologic differences in the behavior of proximal and distal CRC.

USING ADMINISTRATIVE DATA FOR MEASUREMENT OF INDIVIDUAL PHYSICIAN QUALITY OF CARE: THE CENTERS FOR MEDICARE AND MEDICAID SERVICES EXAMPLE

In 2007, the Centers for Medicare and Medicaid Services (CMS) initiated the Physician Quality Reporting Initiative (PQRI).[25] In this program, quality measures are suggested by measure development organizations, such as the National Quality Forum or the American Medical Association Physician Consortium for Performance Improvement,[26] and adopted for implementation using specialized billing codes, registries, or electronic health record reporting. Of 179 measures in the 2010 PQRI measures set, there are 10 individual measures of special interest for gastroenterology and hepatology. Nine of these measures are concerned with hepatitis C. The tenth measure, measure number 185 is titled "Endoscopy & Polyp Surveillance: Colonoscopy Interval for Patients with a History of Adenomatous Polyps – Avoidance of Inappropriate Use" and can be reported using claims data or through a registry. In addition, 8 of the 9 hepatitis C measures can be reported as a group measure.

Providers or group practices that are paid by Medicare through the Physician Fee Schedule program for Part B claims are eligible to participate in this voluntary program. Data is reported each time a surveillance colonoscopy is performed using standard Medicare billing processes. A provider must report on greater than or equal to 80% of applicable patients for each measure to be eligible for incentive payment. To be eligible for submitting measures through a registry, a provider must report on greater than or equal to 3 individual measures or at least 1 measure group.

Measures consist of a numerator and denominator. The denominator identifies the eligible population through CPT Category I codes, Healthcare Common Procedure Coding System G codes (Healthcare Common Procedure Coding System), ICD-9-CM codes, or patient demographics. The numerator identifies the clinical action that is required by the measure and is reported using specialized codes including CPT Category II codes or G codes, which may have modifiers for excluding the case from the denominator. These are specialized codes that are not used otherwise as billing codes; current billing codes without these specialized extensions are not adequate for measuring quality. Measure number 185 illustrates these components. The denominator of this measure is all patients aged 18 years and older receiving a surveillance colonoscopy with a history of colonic polyps in a previous colonoscopy. Criteria include the following, which must be documented in billing to CMS:

- Patients aged 18 years or older on date of encounter AND
- Diagnosis for history of colonic polyps, documented using code V12.72 AND
- Patient encounter during the reporting period, documented using one of the following codes 44388, 44389, 44392, 44393, 44394, 45355, 45378, 45380, 45381, 45383, 45384, 45385, or G0105
- But WITHOUT using CPT Category I modifiers: 52, 53, 73, 74.

The numerator of the measure is patients who had an interval of 3 or more years since their last colonoscopy. Criteria for the numerator include the following:

- Interval of 3 or more years since patients' last colonoscopy, which is reported using the specialized CPT II code 0529F, OR
- Interval of less than 3 years since patients' last colonoscopy for medical or system reasons, reported by appending 0529F with one of the following codes:
    1P: if there is documentation of medical reasons for an interval less than 3 years (eg, patients at high risk for colon cancer, last colonoscopy

incomplete, last colonoscopy had inadequate prep, piecemeal removal of adenomas, or last colonoscopy found >10 adenomas),

3P: if there is documentation of system reasons for an interval of less than 3 years (eg, unable to locate previous colonoscopy report), or

8P: if the reason is not specified.

At least one other PQRI measure may be of interest to all providers. Measure number 124 (Health Information Technology, Adoption/Use of Electronic Health Records ([EHR]) documents whether the provider has adopted and is using health information technology. To qualify, the provider must have adopted and be using a certified/qualified EHR.

Success of the CMS PQRI program is unknown and no published studies could be found demonstrating enhancement of quality based on the PQRI program. It is reasonable to believe, however, that performance feedback can be effective even without payment for that performance.[27–29] At the time of this writing, the CMS-proposed rule has been published for implementation of the meaningful use provisions of the HITECH (Health Information Technology for Economic and Clinical Health) Act.[30] The effect on the PQRI program is yet to be determined.

COMPLETENESS AND ACCURACY OF DATA IN CLINICAL REGISTRIES

Data derived from disease registries or health surveys avoid many of the biases noted with administrative data. Quality of data, however, remains an issue, although the expectations for these data sources are high. Arts and colleagues[31] described a framework of procedures for assuring data quality in medical registries (**Table 1**) that takes into account the 2 methods of data collection, automated extraction from electronic records, and manual abstraction of data from paper or electronic records. In a case study on measurement errors, they analyzed registry data from 2 intensive care units contributing to the same registry. Regardless of the method used, the registry data was found to contain inaccuracies (2.0% of the time for electronic vs 4.6% for manual data extraction) and missing elements (4.0% for electronic and 5.0% for manual data extraction). A significant difference between the 2 methods is that when data is automatically extracted from electronic systems, data errors tend to be systematic rather than random, as seen with manual data extraction, and therefore error rates can be lowered with correction of programming errors.

Black and Payne[32] have also developed a quality checklist for clinical registries (**Table 2**) expressing conformance to 10 criteria representing completeness and accuracy of registry data. They later used self-reported data and some of these criteria to measure the quality of data in 105 registries in the United Kingdom.[33] Many of these registries were used for ad hoc analyses for providers, or for audit reports, but 75% previously had resulted in papers published in peer review journals, illustrating the power of such registries for multiple purposes.

As part of its Effective Health Care Program, the Agency for Healthcare Research and Quality produced a handbook for use by prospective or established clinical registries performing outcomes research, a handbook that is equally useful for registries designed to enhance quality.[1] The authors of this handbook point out the lack of evidence for quantifiable parameters that either indicate quality of registry data or quality of the conclusions drawn by studies using the data. Given this limitation, they chose to present guidelines for both research quality (ie, quality of the scientific process, such as design and operational aspects of the registry) and evidence quality (ie, quality of the data and findings resulting from the research process).

Table 1
Framework of procedures for the assurance of data quality in medical registries

Central Coordinating Center	Local Sites
Prevention during set up and organization of registry	
At the onset of the registry	*At the onset of participating in the registry*
Compose minimum set of necessary data items	Assign a contact person
Define data and data characteristics in data dictionary	Check developed software for data entry and for extraction
Draft a data collection protocol	Check reliability and completeness of extraction sources
Define pitfalls in data collection	Standardize correction of data items
Compose data checks	*Continuously*
Create user friendly case record forms	Train (new) data collectors
Create quality assurance plan	Motivate data collectors
In case of new participating sites	Make data definitions available
Perform site visit	Place date and initials on completed forms
Train new participants	Keep completed case record forms
Continuously	Data collection close to the source and as soon as possible
Motivate participants	Use the registry data for local purposes
Communicate with local sites	*In case of changes (eg, in data set)*
In case of changes (eg, in data sets)	Adjust data dictionary, forms, software, and so forth
Adjust forms, software, data dictionary, protocol, training material, and so forth	Communicate with data collectors
Communicate with local sites	
Detection during data collection	
During import of data into the central database	Continuously
Perform automatic data checks	Visually inspect completed forms
Periodically and in case of new participants	Perform automatic data checks
Perform site visits for data quality audit (registry data <> source data) and review local data collection procedures	Check completeness of registration
Periodically	
Check interobserver and intraobserver variability	
Perform analyses on the data	
Actions for quality improvement	
After data import and data checks	*After receiving quality reports*
Provide local sites with data quality reports	Check detected errors
Control local correction of data errors	Correct inaccurate data and fill in incomplete data
After data audit or variability test	Resolve causes of data errors
Give feedback of results and recommendations	*After receiving feedback*
Resolve causes of data errors	Implement recommended changes
	Communicate with personnel

From Arts DG, De Keizer NF, Scheffer GJ. Defining and improving data quality in medical registries: a literature review, case study, and generic framework. J Am Med Inform Assoc 2002;9:600.

Table 2
Criteria for assessing the coverage and accuracy of a clinical database (intermediate levels 2 and 3 not shown)

Criteria	Level 1 (Low Compliance)	Level 4 (High Compliance)
Extent to which the eligible population is representative of the country	No evidence or unlikely to be representative	Total population of country included
Completeness of recruitment of eligible population	Few (<80%) or unknown	All or almost all (>97%)
Variables included in the database	Identifier, administrative information, condition, or intervention	Identifier, administrative information, condition, intervention, short-term outcome, major known confounders, long-term outcome
Completeness of data (percentage variables at least 95% complete)	Few (<50% or unknown)	All or almost all (>97%)
Form in which continuous data (excluding dates) are collected (percentage collected as raw data)	Few (<70%) or unknown	All or almost all (>97%) or no continuous data collected
Use of explicit definitions for variables	None	All or almost all (>97%)
Use of explicit rules for deciding how variables are recorded	None	All or almost all (>97%)
Reliability of coding of conditions and interventions	Not tested	Good
Independence of observations of primary outcome	Outcome not included or independence unknown	Independent observer blinded to intervention or not necessary as objective outcome (eg, death or laboratory test)
Extent to which data are validated	No validation	Range and consistency checks plus external validation using alternative source

Adapted from Black N, Payne M. Directory of clinical databases: improving and promoting their use. Qual Saf Health Care 2003;12:348.

Perhaps the most important question to ask here is whether the burden of data collection for clinical registries is too large to assure participation by clinical sites or to assure quality of the data collected. For clinicians, time is of the essence and entering or reentering data that is not specifically needed for documentation and communication of clinical history and findings or for reimbursement is universally resisted. Data abstraction of registry data from medical charts is resource intensive not only for personnel performing the data abstraction but also for registry personnel responsible for training, communication, updates, auditing, and data validation. The processes of the Society of Thoracic Surgeons (STS) national database illustrate this point.

The STS national database supports 4 databases, including the Adult Cardiac Surgery Database, which has been gathering data since 1989 with a primary goal of determining risk-adjusted operative outcomes.[34] This registry is also useful for enhancing quality; from more than 40 published articles since its inception are articles specifically on quality of care. In 2007, the STS initiated a quality measurement program, including individual quality indicators and overall composite scores.[35,36] In addition, since 2009, the STS has been certified to report directly to CMS on 3 PQRI measures. The cost of participation in this program seems high, but despite this burden for data collection, more than 150,000 patient records were submitted in 2007 from 809 hospitals.[37]

Requirements for sites to participate include the following:

- Employment of a data manager (responsible for data entry, extracting data for computerized reports, analyzing reports, checking on data quality, and presentation of results) who should have a clinical background, preferably in a critical care environment, such as a registered nurse or physician assistant
- Purchase or development of certified software with appropriate computing infrastructure and technology assistance at the site
- Payment of participation fees
- Provision of required working space for the data manager and computing infrastructure
- Entry of data by multiple personnel at the point of care (the preferred method) or through chart abstraction (point of care data entry on paper records with later secondary entry into the computer system recommended)
- Submission of data to the data coordinating center twice a year with resubmission as needed until data quality issues are resolved.

For the gastroenterology (GI) community, the GI Quality Improvement Consortium, Ltd[38] is currently developing a national registry that will allow physicians and groups to determine performance on selected quality measures and to benchmark against other participants. Submission of data to the CMS PQRI program is anticipated.

USING ELECTRONIC HEALTH RECORD DATABASES TO ENHANCE QUALITY

With the increasing emphasis on documentation of all clinical activities using electronic health records, the question arises whether or not EHRs can be a source for enhancing quality in an automated fashion, without requiring manual review of clinical records. Even where electronic documentation of clinical episodes is the rule, most notes are dictated narrative with few external standards for content, the exceptions being laboratory results, and medication and problem lists when these are structured or encoded. Narrative reports work extremely well for the primary purpose of documentation; dictation is fast, it is familiar, and dictated reports often follow a common specialty-specific format. Narrative reports document events well and are effective in communications between providers. However, they are not effective in some health information exchange settings, for example, the sharing of a summary patient record or consolidation of medication prescriptions and dispensations across organizations. And narrative is clearly less than optimal for secondary uses of clinical data, such as clinical decision support, administrative decision support, research, and quality measurement.

A main advantage of using the primary clinical documentation for quality research and measurement is that this data is already being collected for clinical care and therefore likely to represent the full spectrum of care for a clinician, group, or health care facility. The main disadvantage is similar to what we have seen with administrative data, that this data is collected for purposes other than for quality measurement and may not meet the high standards required for this and other secondary uses. In clinical documentation, for example, imprecise terminology and missing, and even inconsistent, data may be managed without difficulty by clinicians who have expertise and contextual knowledge, but not well by computers. It is difficult to extract data from unstructured, narrative text, despite the efforts of many research centers to perfect techniques of text processing. Although adding structure to narrative text with controlled sections improves the machine usability without significantly decreasing human usability of clinical reports and reporting systems, it is the capture of well-defined, discrete, and coded data elements that allows full use of clinical data for secondary purposes, including quality research and reporting.

The concepts of using clinical data captured in electronic health records for purposes, such as quality measurement, have been discussed for severa; years,[39–41] but the implementation of systems that use this data alone are still limited and much of the discussion remains in the medical informatics world. Perhaps a mark of maturity of this domain will be when automated extraction of data from EHRs is no longer a topic for publication. Although experience is gaining in the extraction of quality measurement data from EHRs, it is difficult for clinicians who use EHRs in practice to understand why their data is not easily retrieved for these purposes.

Several recent studies have illustrated both the advantages to and difficulties of accessing and interpreting EHR data. When coded problem lists, medication lists, and laboratory results are available, there is evidence that target populations, the denominator of quality measures, can be identified more accurately than with administrative data, and 97% accuracy has been demonstrated for identifying cases with diabetes.[42] Not all EHRs code problem lists, however. In outpatient EHRs, especially, clinicians may not enter diagnoses for acute illnesses in a problem list and coded visit diagnoses may not be available.[43] In addition, coded visit diagnoses are often used for administrative purposes, using the same coding systems and therefore having the same issues with content coverage.

Inability to document elements of quality measurement in a computable fashion may also be a problem with EHRs. This problem was recently demonstrated by Linder and colleagues[43] who used an EHR to identify elements in a community-acquired pneumonia (CAP) performance measure set. Manual extraction of the electronic record for the performance elements needed for the CAP measure set included assessment of the percentage of elements that were available in coded form. Coding of information ranged from 0% for 4 measures (rationale for location of care, chest radiograph performed, hydration status, and mental status) to 100% for documentation of vaccinations and antibiotics. Identification of measure exclusion criteria[44,45] may be especially difficult in EHRs and underreporting may be irregular and difficult to explain.[41] Ability to use EHRs may depend on modification of user interfaces to promote specific data collection[46] or on alternate methods of capturing data, such as through use of clinical reminders.[47]

A potential advantage of EHRs that has not been explored until recently is that they may allow discovery of better quality measures, ones that reflect varying levels of disease severity, and therefore accounting for the fact that although physicians may control processes, outcomes are only partially under the control of physicians. Persell demonstrated use of in-depth clinical data to "distinguish adequate from inadequate care in complex patients," enabling more advanced performance measures.[48]

ELECTRONIC REPORTING SOFTWARE FOR GASTROINTESTINAL ENDOSCOPY: THE CLINICAL OUTCOMES RESEARCH INITIATIVE EXPERIENCE

The Clinical Outcomes Research Initiative (CORI) experience is an example of how endoscopic reporting software may be used to measure and enhance quality. The CORI reporting software was developed to support outcomes research and is currently used by a national consortium of endoscopists to document endoscopic procedures. Data from each procedure is automatically exported to the National Endoscopic Database after removal of individual identifiers. The CORI reporting software captures the majority of data as discrete elements. Design of the structured fields has required careful planning such that options are both exclusive and exhaustive for each field and the goal is to minimize free text while still allowing endoscopists the degree of expression required for clinical documentation.

A 2009 study[49] demonstrated that quality could be measured using this data, but it also demonstrated how, even with a structured reporting system, clinicians often do not enter important quality data. In this study, data sources included 74 practice sites in 24 states, 79% of which were from private practice. This data has previously been shown to be representative of endoscopic practice in the United States.[50] More than 430,000 colonoscopy reports were analyzed. Performance measures studied were derived from recommendations of expert panels (the Multi-Society Task Force on Colorectal Cancer and the National Colorectal Cancer Roundtable).[51,52]

Results are summarized in **Table 3**. The failure to report the quality of bowel prep (missing in 13.9%) and cecal landmarks (14.1%) represent significant reporting deficiencies. Anyone reading a report would be unable to determine the adequacy of the examination without these key elements.

This example highlights some possible ways in which an electronic database may be used to improve quality. The authors' hypothesis is that if endoscopists can measure and monitor quality indicators in their practice with database reports, performance will improve. Therefore, individuals using a database like CORI can measure performance, and produce individual feedback reports, and then monitor practice to determine if quality improves. In addition, CORI can produce reports of pooled data from multiple practice sites to provide comparative, benchmarking data. Individual providers can use these reports to compare their performance with the pooled

Table 3
Documentation of key quality indicators from the CORI consortium

Reporting Indicator	Completion (%)
Procedure indication	100.0[a]
ASA classification of comorbidity	89.9
Quality of bowel prep recorded	86.1
Report of cecal landmarks	85.9
Polyp descriptors	
Polyp size	95.0
Morphology (sessile, pedunculated, flat)	85.3
Retrieval for pathology reported	95.5

Abbreviation: ASA, American Society of Anesthesiologists.
[a] A mandatory field.
From Lieberman DA, Faigel DO, Logan JR, et al. Assessment of the quality of colonoscopy reports: results from a multicenter consortium. Gastrointest Endosc 2009;69:645.

results. These hypotheses are currently under study, and the authors expect that performance will gradually improve with individual and pooled group feedback.

CURRENT CHALLENGES IN THE USE OF EHR DATA FOR ENHANCING QUALITY

When Data is Unstructured: Natural Language Processing

Most clinical documentation is at the other end of the documentation spectrum from the CORI model, that is, captured in narrative text. Algorithms for processing this text, resulting in identification of clinical concepts that can then be used for quality measurement and research, are an active area of research. Domains that have been studied include radiology,[53] vaccine adverse events,[54] and pathology reports.[55] Prominent recognition problems, for example, are the negation of concepts (history of adenomatous polyps vs *no* history of adenomatous polyps) and establishment of context (indication for procedure of reflux symptoms vs past history of reflux symptoms). Clinical text that is readily understood by clinicians may be readily misunderstood by computers.

Regulatory and Ethical Issues

For a recent and insightful discussion of regulatory and ethical issues in quality assessment and improvement activities, with the STS National Database as a case study, see the article from Dokholyan and colleagues.[56] The primary controversy concerns the need for Institutional Review Board scrutiny of quality improvement processes.

The Standardization of the Language of Medicine: Terminology, Document Architecture, and Interoperability

As a final note on the use of EHRs in quality research and measurement, a mention of emerging standards and initiatives is in order. We are still in the middle of the "Decade of Health Information Technology" declared in 2004[57] and will soon be implementing the HITECH Act proposals.[30] For a description of the structure of EHRs in this environment and how they can contribute to GI research, see Atreja and colleagues.[58] But implementation of EHRs only satisfies part of data needs for enhancing quality; the other need is for standardization of the structure of EHR clinical and quality reporting documents, of terminologies used, and of methods of communication between information systems for quality measurement. Public and private initiatives are contributing to the converging efforts for these standards.

This is an exciting time for health care information technology professionals, but a demanding time for clinicians. Meaningful use, pay for performance, and certification requirements will drive specific quality improvement programs. Registries and electronic health records must evolve to provide clinicians a way to participate in quality research and measurement and quality improvement efforts during demanding clinical practices.

SUMMARY

Administrative databases, registries, and clinical databases are designed for different purposes and therefore have different advantages and disadvantages in providing data for enhancing quality. Administrative databases provide the advantages of size, availability, and generalizability, but are subject to constraints inherent in the coding systems used and from data-collection methods optimized for billing. Registries are designed for research and quality reporting, but require significant investment from participants for secondary data collection and quality control. Electronic health records contain all of the data needed for quality research and measurement, but that data is too often locked in narrative text and unavailable for analysis. National mandates for electronic health record implementation and functionality will likely change this landscape in the near future.

REFERENCES

1. (Prepared by Outcome dEcIDE Center [Outcome Sciences, Inc dba Outcome] under Contract No. HHSA29020050035[T01]. AHRQ Publication No. 07-EHC001-1). In: Gliklich RE, Dreyer NA, editors. Registries for evaluating patient outcomes: a user's guide. Rockville (MD): Agency for Healthcare Research and Quality; April 2007. Available at: http://www.effectivehealthcare. ahrq.gov. Accessed January 28, 2010.
2. LOINC: Logical Observation Identifiers Names and Codes. Regenstrief Institute, Inc; 2010. Available at: http://loinc.org. Accessed February 22, 2010.
3. Huff SM, Rocha RA, McDonald CJ, et al. Development of the Logical Observation Identifier Names and Codes (LOINC) vocabulary. J Am Med Inform Assoc 1998; 5:276.
4. Khan AN, Griffith SP, Moore C, et al. Standardizing laboratory data by mapping to LOINC. J Am Med Inform Assoc 2006;13:353.
5. Davila JA, El-Serag HB. GI Epidemiology: databases for epidemiological studies. Aliment Pharmacol Ther 2007;25:169.
6. Everhart JE, editor. The burden of digestive diseases in the United States. U.S. Department of Health and Human Services, Public Health Service, National Institutes of Health, National Institute of Diabetes and Digestive and Kidney Diseases. Washington, DC: U.S. Government Printing Office; 2008. NIH Publication No. 09–6443.
7. Richter JE. The enormous burden of digestive diseases on our healthcare system. Curr Gastroenterol Rep 2003;5:93.
8. Sandler RS, Everhart JE, Donowitz M, et al. The burden of selected digestive diseases in the United States. Gastroenterology 2002;122:1500.
9. Shaheen NJ, Hansen RA, Morgan DR, et al. The burden of gastrointestinal and liver diseases, 2006. Am J Gastroenterol 2006;101:2128.
10. National Healthcare Quality Report 2008. AHRQ Publication No. 07-EHC001-1. Rockville (MD): Agency for Healthcare Research and Quality; March 2009. Available at: http://www.ahrq.gov/qual/nhqr08/nhqr08.pdf. Accessed February 14, 2010.
11. NQF-Endorsed Standards. The National Quality Forum. Available at: http://www. qualityforum.org/Measures_List.aspx. Accessed February 25, 2010.
12. Clancy C. The performance of performance measurement. Health Serv Res 2007; 42:1797.
13. Black C, Roos NP. Administrative data. Baby or bathwater? Med Care 1998;36:3.
14. Iezzoni LI. Assessing quality using administrative data. Ann Intern Med 1997;127: 666.
15. Iezzoni LI. Finally present on admission but needs attention. Med Care 2007;45: 280.
16. Mohammed MA, Stevens A. The value of administrative databases. BMJ 2007; 334:1014.
17. Jollis JG, Ancukiewicz M, DeLong ER, et al. Discordance of databases designed for claims payment versus clinical information systems. Implications for outcomes research. Ann Intern Med 1993;119:844.
18. Keating NL, Landrum MB, Landon BE, et al. Measuring the quality of diabetes care using administrative data: is there bias? Health Serv Res 2003;38:1529.

19. Solberg LI, Engebretson KI, Sperl-Hillen JM, et al. Are claims data accurate enough to identify patients for performance measures or quality improvement? The case of diabetes, heart disease, and depression. Am J Med Qual 2006;21:238.

20. Davenport DL, Holsapple CW, Conigliaro J. Assessing surgical quality using administrative and clinical data sets: a direct comparison of the University HealthSystem Consortium Clinical Database and the National Surgical Quality Improvement Program data set. Am J Med Qual 2009;24:395.

21. University HealthSystem Consortium. University HealthSystem Consortium. 2010. Available at: https://www.uhc.edu./. Accessed March 6, 2010.

22. About ACS NSQIP. American College of Surgeons National Quality Improvement Program. 2006. Available at: https://acsnsqip.org/main/about_overview.asp. Accessed March 6, 2010.

23. Baxter NN, Goldwasser MA, Paszat LF, et al. Association of Colonoscopy and Death from Colorectal Cancer. Ann Intern Med 2009;150:1–8.

24. Winawer SJ, Zauber AG, Ho MN, et al. Prevention of colorectal cancer by colonoscopic polypectomy. The National Polyp Study Workgroup. N Engl J Med 1993; 329:1977.

25. Physicians Quality Reporting Initiative (PQRI). U.S. Department of Health & Human Services, Centers for Medicare and Medicaid Services. Available at: http://www.cms.hhs.gov/pqrip. November 18 2009. Accessed March 6, 2010.

26. Physician Consortium for Performance Improvement (PCPI). American Medical Association. 2010. Available at: http://www.ama-assn.org/ama/pub/physician-resources/clinical-practice-improvement/clinical-quality/physician-consortium-performanace-improvement.shtml. Accessed March 6, 2010.

27. Jamtvedt G, Young JM, Kristoffersen DT, et al. Does telling people what they have been doing change what they do? A systematic review of the effects of audit and feedback. Qual Saf Health Care 2006;15:433–6.

28. Walsh JME, McDonald KM, Shojania KG, et al. Quality improvement strategies for hypertension management: a systematic review. Med Care 2006;44(7):646–57.

29. Chaillet N, Dubé E, Dugas M, et al. Evidence-based strategies for implementing guidelines in obstetrics: a systematic review. Obstet Gynecol 2006;108:1234–45.

30. Health Information Technology for Economic and Clinical Health Act (HITECH Act), Title XIII of Division A and Title IV of Division B of the American Recovery and Reinvestment Act, (ARRA) Section 4101, Pub Law No. 111–5, (2009).

31. Arts DG, De Keizer NF, Scheffer GJ. Defining and improving data quality in medical registries: a literature review, case study, and generic framework. J Am Med Inform Assoc 2002;9:600.

32. Black N, Payne M. Directory of clinical databases: improving and promoting their use. Qual Saf Health Care 2003;12:348.

33. Black N, Barker M, Payne M. Cross sectional survey of multicentre clinical databases in the United Kingdom. BMJ 2004;328:1478.

34. Ferguson TB Jr, Dziuban SW Jr, Edwards FH, et al. The STS National Database: current changes and challenges for the new millennium. Committee to Establish a National Database in Cardiothoracic Surgery, The Society of Thoracic Surgeons. Ann Thorac Surg 2000;69:680.

35. O'Brien SM, Shahian DM, DeLong ER, et al. Quality measurement in adult cardiac surgery: part 2–Statistical considerations in composite measure scoring and provider rating. Ann Thorac Surg 2007;83:S13.

36. Shahian DM, Edwards FH, Ferraris VA, et al. Quality measurement in adult cardiac surgery: part 1–Conceptual framework and measure selection. Ann Thorac Surg 2007;83:S3.

37. Shahian DM, O'Brien SM, Normand SL, et al. Association of hospital coronary artery bypass volume with processes of care, mortality, morbidity, and the Society of Thoracic Surgeons composite quality score. J Thorac Cardiovasc Surg 2010; 139:273.
38. GI Quality Improvement Project Description. GI Quality Improvement Consortium, Ltd. Available at: http://www.giquic.org/description.asp. Accessed March 6, 2010.
39. Einbinder JS, Scully K. Using a clinical data repository to estimate the frequency and costs of adverse drug events. Proc AMIA Symp 2001;154.
40. McDonald CJ, Overhage JM, Dexter P, et al. A framework for capturing clinical data sets from computerized sources. Ann Intern Med 1997;127:675.
41. Owen RR, Thrush CR, Cannon D, et al. Use of electronic medical record data for quality improvement in schizophrenia treatment. J Am Med Inform Assoc 2004; 11:351.
42. Tang PC, Ralston M, Arrigotti MF, et al. Comparison of methodologies for calculating quality measures based on administrative data versus clinical data from an electronic health record system: implications for performance measures. J Am Med Inform Assoc 2007;14:10.
43. Linder JA, Kaleba EO, Kmetik KS. Using electronic health records to measure physician performance for acute conditions in primary care: empirical evaluation of the community-acquired pneumonia clinical quality measure set. Med Care 2009;47:208.
44. Baker DW, Persell SD, Thompson JA, et al. Automated review of electronic health records to assess quality of care for outpatients with heart failure. Ann Intern Med 2007;146:270.
45. Persell SD, Wright JM, Thompson JA, et al. Assessing the validity of national quality measures for coronary artery disease using an electronic health record. Arch Intern Med 2006;166:2272.
46. O'Toole MF, Kmetik KS, Bossley H, et al. Electronic health record systems: the vehicle for implementing performance measures. Am Heart Hosp J 2005;3:88.
47. Goulet JL, Erdos J, Kancir S, et al. Measuring performance directly using the veterans health administration electronic medical record: a comparison with external peer review. Med Care 2007;45:73.
48. Persell SD, Kho AN, Thompson JA, et al. Improving hypertension quality measurement using electronic health records. Med Care 2009;47:388.
49. Lieberman DA, Faigel DO, Logan JR, et al. Assessment of the quality of colonoscopy reports: results from a multicenter consortium. Gastrointest Endosc 2009; 69:645.
50. Sonnenberg A, Amorosi SL, Lacey MJ, et al. Patterns of endoscopy in the United States: analysis of data from the Centers for Medicare and Medicaid Services and the National Endoscopic Database. Gastrointest Endosc 2008;67:489.
51. Lieberman D, Nadel M, Smith RA, et al. Standardized colonoscopy reporting and data system: report of the Quality Assurance Task Group of the National Colorectal Cancer Roundtable. Gastrointest Endosc 2007;65:757.
52. Rex DK, Bond JH, Winawer S, et al. Quality in the technical performance of colonoscopy and the continuous quality improvement process for colonoscopy: recommendations of the U.S. Multi-Society Task Force on Colorectal Cancer. Am J Gastroenterol 2002;97:1296.
53. Hripcsak G, Friedman C, Alderson PO, et al. Unlocking clinical data from narrative reports: a study of natural language processing. Ann Intern Med 1995;122: 681.

54. Hazlehurst B, Naleway A, Mullooly J. Detecting possible vaccine adverse events in clinical notes of the electronic medical record. Vaccine 2009;27:2077.

55. D'Avolio LW, Litwin MS, Rogers SO Jr, et al. Facilitating Clinical Outcomes Assessment through the automated identification of quality measures for prostate cancer surgery. J Am Med Inform Assoc 2008;15:341.

56. Dokholyan RS, Muhlbaier LH, Falletta JM, et al. Regulatory and ethical considerations for linking clinical and administrative databases. Am Heart J 2009;157:971.

57. The Decade of Health Information Technology: delivering consumer-centric and information-rich health care. Framework for Strategic Action. Tommy G. Thompson, Secretary of Health and Human Services and David G. Brailer, National Coordinator for Health Information Technology. July 21, 2004.

58. Atreja A, Achkar JP, Jain AK, et al. Using technology to promote gastrointestinal outcomes research: a case for electronic health records. Am J Gastroenterol 2008;103:2171.

Defining an Episode of Care for Colonoscopy: Work of the High Value Health Care Project Characterizing Episodes and Costs of Care

Niall J. Brennan, MPP[a], Todd A. Lee, PharmD, PhD[b,c,d,*], Adam S. Wilk, BA[a], Christopher S. Lyttle, MA[e], Kevin B. Weiss, MD[f]

KEYWORDS

- Colonoscopy • Resource use • Episode

Numerous studies have indicated that the United States spends significantly more per person on health care than any other nation in the world. Additionally, research has documented significant variation in spending by provider and by region in the United States and that this variation often has little or no correlation with the quality of care provided or with patient outcomes.[1,2] Although reducing health care spending is a central goal of the health care reform debate, clear evidence on the best ways to do so remains out of reach.

This work was supported by Grant No. 63609 from the Robert Wood Johnson Foundation. The authors have nothing to disclose.

[a] Engelberg Center for Health Care Reform, The Brookings Institution, 1775 Massachusetts Avenue, NW, Washington, DC 20036, USA

[b] Center for Management of Complex Chronic Care, Hines VA Hospital, 5000 South 5th Avenue, Building 1, B-260, Hines, IL 60141, USA

[c] Department of Pharmacy Practice, Center for Pharmacoeconomics Research, University of Illinois at Chicago, 833 South Wood Street, Chicago, IL 60612, USA

[d] Department of Pharmacy Administration, Center for Pharmacoeconomics Research, University of Illinois at Chicago, 833 South Wood Street, Chicago, IL 60612, USA

[e] Institute for Healthcare Studies, Northwestern University, 750 North Lake Shore Drive, 10th Floor, Chicago, IL 60611, USA

[f] American Board of Medical Specialties Research and Education Foundation, 222 North LaSalle Street, Suite 1500, Chicago, IL 60601, USA

* Corresponding author. Center for Management of Complex Chronic Care, Hines VA Hospital, 5000 South 5th Avenue, Building 1, B-260, Hines, IL 60141.
E-mail address: niall.brennan@cms.hhs.gov

Gastrointest Endoscopy Clin N Am 20 (2010) 735–750
doi:10.1016/j.giec.2010.07.014
1052-5157/10/$ – see front matter. Published by Elsevier Inc.

Although documentation of variability in the overall costs of care at regional levels points out that inefficiencies exist in the health care system, it does not provide actionable information on what may be the underlying cause of the differences and how these differences can be reduced. One potential solution is to focus on episode-based resource use and costs so that differences within a particular clinical area can be examined and areas in need of action can be identified. Moreover, episode-based measures may be combined with quality of care measures to provide some insights in identifying efficient care in which quality is high and costs are low. Such information would allow all parties involved (consumers, purchasers, and providers) to better understand how treatment decisions affect the costs and quality of their care. Data gathered from such analyses have the potential to provide clear and actionable information on what components of care can (or should) be reduced and what components of care can (or should) be increased, thereby helping to reduce spending while at the same time maintaining or even improving clinical quality and outcomes.[3,4]

Ideally, in order for a given condition or procedure to be a candidate for an episode-based measure of health care costs, a clear body of evidence that supports the relevant clinical management and treatment decisions should be readily available. The use of colonoscopy in colon cancer screening is one of these areas highly suitable for such episode-based measure development. We have developed an episode-based measure of costs of care associated with screening colonoscopy, and our subsequent analytic findings of the measure suggest that it can serve as a helpful tool for identifying, and potentially addressing, unwarranted variability in resource use related to the performance of such procedures.

Colorectal cancer is one of the most commonly diagnosed cancers in the United States. In 2005, more than 140,000 men and women were diagnosed with colorectal cancer, and approximately 52,000 died from of the condition.[5] Both the Institute of Medicine and the Ambulatory Care Quality Alliance (AQA) have identified colon cancer as 1 of 20 condition-specific priority areas in need of quality improvement, based on its relevance to a considerable volume of patients, its impact on those patients, and the perception of opportunity to significantly improve the quality and efficiency of related care.[6] The complete list of priority condition-specific areas is included as follows.

- Acute Myocardial Infarction
- Angina/Coronary Artery Disease
- Asthma
- Breast Cancer
- Bronchitis
- Chronic Obstructive Pulmonary Disease
- Colon Cancer
- Congestive Heart Failure
- Depression
- Diabetes
- Hiatal Hernia (Gastroesophageal Reflux Disease)
- Hip Fracture
- Hypertension
- Hysterectomy
- Low Back Pain
- Osteoarthritis
- Pneumonia
- Prostate Cancer

- Sinusitis
- Stroke.

Colorectal cancer screening has been shown to reduce colorectal cancer mortality by as much as 60%.[7,8] Although there are a variety of ways to screen for colorectal cancer, the most popular method used today is colonoscopy. This procedure involves the insertion through the rectum of a flexible videoscope, which is then advanced proximally through the entire length of the colon to search for the presence of polyps.[9] Colonoscopy is the preferred colorectal cancer screening strategy of both the American College of Gastroenterology (ACG) and the American Society of Colon and Rectal Surgeons (ASCRS), receiving a Grade 1B recommendation in the ACG's most recent guidelines (issued in 2008).[10] Colon cancer screening is similarly recommended by the US Preventive Services Task Force and has also been identified as a priority area in other national initiatives, including the Health Resources and Services Administration's (HRSA) Health Disparities Collaboratives and the Centers for Medicare and Medicaid Services' (CMS) Quality Improvement Program.[11]

Although the role of colonoscopy in detecting and preventing colon cancer is clear, concerns have been raised in recent years about the overall rising costs of the procedure. These concerns are in part based on the increasing total volume of colonoscopy procedures performed as well as the increasing costs of each individual procedure. In 2003, for example, 30% of eligible women and 32% of eligible men 50 years and older had undergone the procedure.[12,13] The rising costs of each procedure may largely be attributable to increasing costs of ancillary resources that are used. For example, because patient discomfort during the procedure can be considerable, some sort of sedation or anesthesia is typically administered. However, the type of sedation given, whether or not more complete anesthesia should be used, and whether or not sedation is even necessary at all in every circumstance is of some debate. As a result, considerable individual provider discretion is the norm.[14] Furthermore, the procedure has some inherently associated potential complications (eg, bleeding and bowel perforation), and the potential for these complications to occur may also vary depending on the level of sedation. Whereas procedures performed with sedation have higher risks of respiratory depression, falls, and other sedation-related complications, those performed without sedation have higher failure rates in part because of patient discomfort.[15–17]

MEASURING RESOURCE USE AND COSTS OF CARE

Alternative methodologies exist that can be used to measure the resource use associated with a colonoscopic examination and individual health care costs in general. The 2 primary approaches are per-capita measurement and per-episode measurement. Per-capita measurement captures the cumulative health care costs for a given population. Examples of this methodology include measures of total costs per member per month (PMPM) and measures of service use per 1000 patients per year. Although this methodology is relatively easy to implement and interpret, the measures themselves are population-level measures, and accurately establishing and assigning accountability for such population-level measures can be difficult. One reason for this difficulty is the dispersed nature of the medical care that many patients receive. Researchers have found that because many patients see multiple providers for multiple conditions over the course of a given year, assigning meaningful accountability for the total costs of their care can be problematic.[18]

Per-episode measurement quantifies the services involved in the diagnosis, management, and treatment of unique clinical conditions. These measures can capture the total costs associated with any acute or chronic condition of interest. Episode-based measures can also be more focused and precise—as in the case of the colonoscopy measure we describe later in this article. This particular episode-based measure focuses on the patient's preparation before the colonoscopy, the procedure itself, and any related complications following the procedure. Any postprocedure patient management or treatment that may be related to a newly established diagnosis, however, would not be included here; such patient management or treatment could potentially be included in other measurement efforts. Although significantly more complex to develop than per-capita measures, episode-based measures have the advantage of increased clinical specificity and are potentially much more actionable for providers and consumers.

Although commercial vendors currently offer tools that rely on per-episode measurement structures to generate estimates of physician performance based on cost (most prominently Ingenix's Episode Treatment Groups[19] and Thomson-Reuters' Medical Episode Grouper[20]), early efforts to implement these tools have experienced only limited success. Key issues affecting these implementation efforts have included a lack of transparency in the measurement methodologies, inconsistent or ineffective communication with patients and providers during the implementation process, and provider resistance to cost-of-care measurement in any form.[21]

The High Value Health Care (HVHC) Project, funded by the Robert Wood Johnson Foundation and overseen by the Quality Alliance Steering Committee (QASC), is working to make valid, timely, and consistent information about the quality and cost of health care widely available in the United States through furthering the development and use of a performance measurement infrastructure. One component of this effort specifically focuses on the development of a fully transparent set of cost-of-care measures developed with the input and clinical guidance of key stakeholders (including practicing physicians). The goal of structuring the measure development process in this way is to alleviate many of the concerns providers have expressed about other, less transparent, cost-of-care measurement algorithms, such as the proprietary efforts cited previously.[a]

Under this component of the HVHC project called Characterizing Episodes and Cost of Care (C3), the American Board of Medical Specialties Research and Education Foundation (ABMS REF), in conjunction with The Brookings Institution, undertook the development of episode-based cost-of-care measures for 12 of the most prevalent and important acute and chronic conditions in the United States that were identified by the AQA.[6]

Here, we discuss the process by which an episode-based measure of the costs of care associated with colonoscopy has been developed as part of the C3 project and show some of the effort's preliminary analytic findings.

BUILDING AN EPISODE OF CARE FOR COLONOSCOPY

For each of the 12 high-priority conditions included in the HVHC Project, a group of expert clinicians and other stakeholders was convened for a 2-day in-person meeting followed by a series of teleconference meetings. During the in-person meeting, the workgroup focused initially on conceptually defining one or more important measures for the condition, reaching a broad consensus on the cohort definition (including which patients should be excluded from the measure). Then the work group sought to

---

[a] More information regarding the HVHC cost-of-care measure development effort can be found here: http://www.healthqualityalliance.org/hvhc-project/cost-care-measurement-development.

identify the services and resource use that were "related" to the clinical condition of interest for each measure. In this context, "related" services and resource use were defined as all of the medical care provided with the intent of treating or managing the clinical condition of interest as well as all of the care involved in the management of any resulting complications. Notably, this definition does not distinguish any care that is appropriate from any care that is not, nor does it distinguish any care that is in compliance with generally accepted clinical treatment guidelines from care that is not. Relative to the colonoscopy episode, "related" resource use consists of all the care pertinent to the performance of the examination (eg, the procedure itself, sedatives and other medications, attendant supervision), any immediate preparations for the procedure (eg, the bowel preparations, other medications), and any pertinent conditions that may arise in the immediate postprocedure period (eg, bowel perforations, bleeding, repeat colonoscopies).

Following the in-person meeting, the concepts were translated into detailed measure specifications for further review by the clinician work groups. The measure specifications were then developed into a series of computer algorithms and tested using a large administrative claims dataset, benchmark statistics from national research organizations, and pertinent information from the clinical literature.[b] The variability of costs across regions and provider specialties associated with the episode or episodes developed through this process was examined to determine whether each measure was effective in identifying unwarranted variation in costs (ie, variation not attributable to underlying variation in patient complexity or morbidity).

Through this process, a measure was developed that focuses on variation in resource use observed in the 22-day period surrounding a screening colonoscopic examination with the clinical input of the colon cancer clinical work group; primarily methodological input was also provided by the C3 Project's Technical Advisory Committee and the QASC's Episodes Workgroup. The measure includes the resources used during a 7-day period preceding the colonoscopy, those used on the day of the examination, and those used during a 14-day period following the procedure. Members of the work group anticipated that some variability might be observed in the measure's resource use across episodes both as a result of the type of colonoscopy performed (eg, no biopsies, biopsies or polypectomies) and as a result of the types of ancillary services used (eg, no sedation, conscious sedation, or general anesthesia). Additional variation might be seen if there were complications (eg, antibiotics and other medications, lab tests, radiographic examinations, corrective surgical procedures) or if there was a need to repeat the colonoscopy examination itself.[22] Work group members felt that such complication-related resource use would most likely be captured during the 2-week period immediately following the procedure.

COLONOSCOPY EPISODE-OF-CARE COHORT DEFINITION

Accurately defining the population of interest is critical to identifying meaningful variation in resource use for any condition's treatment. Although it may seem a straightforward choice to capture all colonoscopies in a given year, this approach

---

[b] The dataset used for these analyses was the MarketScan Commercial Claims & Encounters Database provided by Thomson Reuters (Healthcare), Inc. The MarketScan data contain claims information for a large population of individuals aged 0 to 64 who were enrolled in a commercial insurance plan during the calendar year 2006 or 2007. In total, the data reflect the health care experience of approximately 15 million covered lives per year. Although all regions of the United States are represented, patients in the database are disproportionately from the South.

can lead to the inclusion of individuals who receive colonoscopies for reasons other than the early detection of colon cancer. Doing so could introduce confounding variability in resource use into the measure. For this and other related reasons, the clinicians participating in the measure development elected to define the colonoscopy measure's eligible population as follows.

Inclusion Criteria

Patients are included in the measure if they had a colonoscopy billed using any of the codes listed in **Table 1** during the 22-day period covered by the episode and if they are 40 years or older at the time of the procedure.[c] As **Table 1** illustrates, CPT code 45378 (Colonoscopy, flexible, proximal to splenic flexure; diagnostic, with or without collection of specimen[s] by brushing or washing, with or without colon decompression [separate procedure]) accounts for 46% of all colonoscopies in our sample, followed by CPT code 45380 (Colonoscopy, with biopsy, single or multiple) which represents 28% of colonoscopies in our sample. Of the remaining types of colonoscopy, only CPT 45385 (Colonoscopy with removal of tumor[s], polyp[s], or other lesion[s] by snare techniques) accounts for more than 10% of cases.

Table 1
Frequency of triggering colonoscopy codes for colonoscopy episode of care

Description	CPT/HCPCS	Frequency	Percent
Colonoscopy, flexible, proximal to splenic flexure; diagnostic, with or without collection of specimen(s) by brushing or washing, with or without colon decompression (separate procedure)	45378	368,860	46%
Colonoscopy, with biopsy, single or multiple	45380	220,663	28%
Colonoscopy, with ablation of tumor(s), polyp(s), or other lesion(s) not amenable to removal by hot biopsy forceps, bipolar cautery, or snare techniques	45383	12,259	2%
Colonoscopy, with removal of tumor(s), polyp(s), or other lesion(s) by hot biopsy or forceps or bipolar cautery	45384	51,448	6%
Colonoscopy, with removal of tumor(s), polyp(s), or other lesion(s) by snare techniques	45385	121,146	15%
Colorectal cancer screening; colonoscopy on individual at high risk	G0105	8,125	1%
Colorectal cancer screening; colonoscopy on individual not meeting criteria for high risk	G0121	15,845	2%
Total		798,346	100%

The data presented precede exclusions for methodological or clinical reasons.

---

[c] We acknowledge that the existing clinical guidelines for colonoscopy recommend screening only for those aged 50 years and older (45 years for African Americans); however, it was the opinion of the clinical expert panel that there are many patients who undergo screening before age 50, usually because of a family history of colon cancer. Additionally, resource use for colonoscopy was not expected to differ significantly by age.

Although **Table 1** illustrates the total number of colonoscopies that can be identified in our data, a number of exclusions need to be made to reach a final analytic sample. These exclusions are made both for methodological and clinical reasons.

Methodological Exclusion Criteria

Because of the fragmented nature of health insurance coverage in the United States, many people, including those with commercial insurance and those with Medicaid coverage, can experience frequent changes in health insurance status. These changes can occur for reasons such as an employment change or, in the case of Medicaid, a loss of eligibility, which is generally calculated on a month-to-month basis. These breaks in coverage pose a major challenge from a measurement perspective because noncontinuous health insurance coverage leads to missing data, making it impossible to accurately calculate either quality- or cost-of-care measures in this population. For example, suppose an individual with diabetes has insurance coverage from January to June of a given year and is uninsured from July to December. In this case, any performance measure spanning more than a 6-month time period will have insufficient data for calculation. Likewise, patients are excluded from the HVHC colonoscopy measure if they did not have medical and prescription drug coverage throughout the measurement window.

Clinical Exclusion Criteria

As discussed previously, one of the key goals of cost-of-care measurement is to quantify and assess *unwarranted* variation in costs. As such, it is important to identify a relatively homogeneous population to which the measure is most applicable and that will not have systematically different health care use because of coexisting conditions. Therefore, active cancer, end-stage renal disease (ESRD), organ transplantation, and HIV/AIDS are routinely used as exclusion criteria for many quality and cost-of-care measures (like the National Committee for Quality Assurance's [NCQA's] Healthcare Effectiveness Data and Information Set [HEDIS] measures, as noted in **Fig. 1**) because of the impact these conditions have on patients' health care use overall. In addition, the colon cancer clinical work group recommended the exclusion of patients with ulcerative colitis, Crohn's disease, or inflammatory bowel disease from the measure because these conditions can lead to colonoscopy procedures that would not be done for colorectal cancer screening. These conditions have different known health care resource use patterns associated with colonoscopy as compared with the general population at large.

Fig. 1 details the impact of the exclusion criteria on the eligible cohort. Although **Fig. 1** identifies almost 800,000 colonoscopies that can be identified during the approximately 11-month identification period[d] using eligible colonoscopy codes, 44% are excluded because of insufficient medical or prescription drug coverage, reducing the number of eligible colonoscopies to slightly less than 450,000.[e] Clinical and demographic exclusions further result in the attrition of an additional 57,126

---

[d] The term "identification period" refers to the period of time during which sufficient data are available both beforehand and afterward to compute the measure using the 2 years of data available for the effort's testing and validation purposes. For the colonoscopy episode, the identification period is January 8, 2007, to December 17, 2007.

[e] It should be noted that requiring 2 years of continuous medical and prescription drug coverage may seem an excessive requirement for a measure of 22 days' duration and unnecessarily limits sample size. We intend to test the sensitivity of our measure results to relaxing the continuous coverage criteria before the conclusion of the project, but for consistency with other measures of a longer duration, we have imposed the same continuous coverage criteria across all measures.

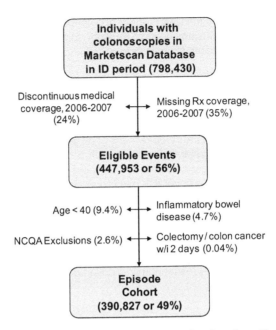

- Note: "inflammatory bowel disease" includes ulcerative colitis, Crohn's disease, and other inflammatory bowel diseases

Fig. 1. Number of colonoscopies in a large claims dataset.

colonoscopies. The final analytic sample consists of 390,827 colonoscopies. Of the clinical and demographic exclusions, those with the largest impact on the measure's denominator are based on age and the presence of inflammatory bowel disease (see **Fig. 1**).

CAPTURING RESOURCE USE RELATED TO COLONOSCOPY

As discussed previously, a key distinguishing characteristic of episode-based measurement methodologies is that they define "related" resource use for a given denominator population over a defined time period. In the case of the colonoscopy measure defined through our process, related resource use and costs are identified in the 7 days before the colonoscopy and in the 14 days following a colonoscopy.

There are several strategies for capturing related resource use for a given condition. The most commonly used strategy is to analyze claims data for occurrences of specific ICD-9 codes that are deemed to be clinically related to the episode of care. For example, the codes for unspecified gastrointestinal hemorrhage (ICD-9 578.9), perforation of the intestine (ICD-9 569.83), and abdominal pain (ICD-9 789.x) were all judged to be clinically related to a colonoscopy, provided they occurred within the episode's measurement window.[f]

---

[f] For a complete list of ICD-9 codes specified as related to colonoscopy, please refer to the measure specification available at the Web site of the Quality Alliance Steering Committee: http://www. healthqualityalliance.org/.

Once all clinically related resource use has been identified, each service is allocated a standard price to ensure that observed differences are a result of variability in provider practice patterns and resource use and are not a result of variations attributable to regional differences in the cost of living or contracted pricing differences.[g] With standard prices applied, all colonoscopy episodes in the sample can be analyzed and compared to see if there is meaningful variation in resource use across episodes and, if so, what specific services drive the observed variations in episode costs.

RESULTS

Table 2 details resource use by type of service for episodes of colonoscopy as calculated using the 2007 MarketScan database. Resource use is broken out into its component parts (ie, by type of service): inpatient facility, outpatient facility, evaluation and management services (E&M), imaging, procedures, tests, prescription drugs, durable medical equipment (DME), and "other services."[h] **Table 2** also details the distribution of costs for each type of service. Average standardized costs for colonoscopy-related services in 2007 were $1192. Unsurprisingly, the 2 dominant type-of-service categories were procedures and outpatient facility costs, comprising 55% and 30% of total colonoscopy episode resource use, respectively. Of the remaining categories of service, only laboratory tests (8%) account for more than 3% of total episode costs.

To evaluate the variability in resource use seen in the colonoscopy episode, we observe that the measure's coefficient of variation is 84% of 85%. As such, compared with episodes of care that have been developed for many other conditions,[i] the overall variation in resource use for episodes of colonoscopy is actually quite modest. However, more significant variability can be observed above the median in per-episode resource use. For example, resource use is 22% higher than the mean ($1455 vs $1192) at the 75th percentile and is 70% higher at the 90th percentile.

Table 3 illustrates the most commonly appearing procedures during these colonoscopy episodes. Among the procedures occurring during these episodes, most are very much as expected, given the codes used to capture colonoscopies for the episode denominator initially. The significance of the anesthesia costs are noteworthy, as are the relatively infrequent but expensive cardiovascular procedures, likely related to complications of the colonoscopy procedure.

---

[g] Standard prices were derived for professional services by calculating mean per-unit costs across all unique Healthcare Common Procedure Coding System (HCPCS) codes and HCPCS modifiers within the MarketScan dataset. Similarly, standard prices for drugs were derived by calculating mean per-day-supply costs within the MarketScan dataset. For inpatient facility costs, the standard prices were based on CMS' per diem costs for each diagnosis-related group (DRG), which were multiplied by the hospital admission's length of stay.

[h] In part, we assign services to type of services categories using the Berenson-Eggers Type of Service (BETOS) Classification system. For more information on the BETOS classification system please refer to http://www.cms.hhs.gov/hcpcsreleasecodesets/20_betos.asp.

[i] The HVHC episodes of asthma (1-year measure of costs associated with the management of asthma), coronary artery disease postrevascularization (1-year management of coronary artery disease following a coronary artery bypass graft [CABG] or percutaneous coronary intervention [PCI] procedure), low back pain with radiculopathy (3-month episode following an office visit with a radiculopathy diagnosis), and community-acquired pneumonia hospitalizations (2-week episode with the patient admitted for pneumonia) saw preliminary median-to-mean cost ratios of 264%, 110%, 263%, and 130%, respectively. Additional information about these other measures is available on the Web site of the Quality Alliance Steering Committee: http://www.healthqualityalliance.org.

Table 2
Distribution of resource use for colonoscopies, by type of service

Description	Mean Costs per Episode	Percent of Total	5th Percentile	10th Percentile	25th Percentile	50th Percentile	75th Percentile	90th Percentile	95th Percentile
Procedures	$658	55.2%	$426	$426	$426	$516	$852	$1056	$1243
Outpatient facility	$359	30.1%	$0	$0	$0	$0	$589	$1077	$1511
Tests	$97	8.1%	$0	$0	$0	$50	$109	$267	$356
Imaging	$25	2.1%	$0	$0	$0	$0	$0	$0	$160
Inpatient facility	$20	1.7%	$0	$0	$0	$0	$0	$0	$0
Drug costs	$16	1.4%	$0	$0	$0	$0	$26	$45	$57
Evaluation and management	$15	1.2%	$0	$0	$0	$0	$0	$0	$65
Other services	$2	0.2%	$0	$0	$0	$0	$0	$0	$0
Durable medical equipment	$0	0.0%	$0	$0	$0	$0	$0	$0	$0
Unclassified	$0	0.0%	$0	$0	$0	$0	$0	$0	$0
Total costs	$1192	100.0%	$426	$426	$625	$1020	$1455	$2030	$2519

Table 3
Frequently occurring procedures for in an episode of colonoscopy

Procedure Code	Description	Total Services	Total Costs
45378	Diagnostic colonoscopy	199,524	$86,805,751
45385	Colonoscopy with removal of tumor, polyp, or lesion by snare technique	81,766	$47,876,659
00810	Anesthesia for lower intestinal endoscopic procedures	120,210	$47,816,403
45380	Colonoscopy with biopsy, single or multiple	94,300	$45,421,491
45384	Colonoscopy with removal of tumor, polyp, or lesion by hot biopsy forceps	31,378	$15,849,063
45383	Colonoscopy with ablation of tumor, polyp, or lesion	7687	$4,483,847
G0105	Colonoscopy on individual at high risk	5001	$1,968,175
43239	Upper GI endoscopy with biopsy, single or multiple	6508	$1,938,227
00902	Anesthesia for anorectal procedure	2790	$1,362,812
00740	Anesthesia for upper IG procedure	1969	$851,864
43235	Diagnostic upper GI endoscopy	2229	$612,813
99144	Moderate sedation services	1029	$114,119
00790	Anesthesia for intraperitoneal procedures in upper abdomen	123	$106,387
00840	Anesthesia for intraperitoneal procedures in lower abdomen	129	$105,431
45382	Colonoscopy with control of bleeding	156	$89,291
44140	Colectomy, partial, with anastomosis	38	$69,036
93510	Left heart catheterization, percutaneous	151	$68,437
92980	Transcatheter placement of an intracoronary stent	38	$51,744
33533	Coronary artery bypass, single arterial graft	21	$42,544
46934	Destruction of hemorrhoids, any method	119	$42,176
Total		559,372	$257,025,768

Approximately three-fourths of the episodes in the final denominator (288,603) showed no claims associated with anesthesia on the date of the colonoscopy, and one-fourth (100,585) showed at least 1 claim associated with general anesthesia on that date.[j] **Table 4** presents resource use by type of service for episodes in these 2 groups, with the costs of anesthesia services and conscious sedation services separated out from the procedures category as presented in **Table 2**. On average, episodes with general anesthesia have 42% higher total costs than episodes with no anesthesia services provided on the day of the colonoscopy ($1523 vs $1075, respectively). Aside from the costs of the anesthesia services themselves, however,

---

[j] The remaining 1420 episodes showed evidence of conscious sedation only during the procedure. This group's resource use was not included in **Table 4** because of its comparatively small sample size.

Table 4
Variation in resource use for colonoscopies, by level of anesthesia

Description	No Anesthesia		General Anesthesia	
	Mean Costs per Episode	Percent of Total	Mean Costs per Episode	Percent of Total
Procedures	$538	50.1%	$513	33.7%
Outpatient facility	$361	33.6%	$347	22.8%
General anesthesia[a]	$2	0.2%	$485	31.9%
Tests	$96	8.9%	$100	6.5%
Imaging	$25	2.3%	$25	1.7%
Inpatient facility	$20	1.9%	$18	1.2%
Drug costs	$16	1.5%	$17	1.1%
Evaluation and management	$15	1.4%	$13	0.9%
Other services	$2	0.2%	$3	0.2%
Durable medical equipment	$0	0.0%	$1	0.0%
Unclassified	$0	0.0%	$0	0.0%
Conscious sedation	$0	0.0%	$0	0.0%
Total costs	$1075	100.0%	$1523	100.0%

[a] "General Anesthesia" group identified based on the presence of general anesthesia services on the date of the colonoscopy defining the episode's measurement window. Other general anesthesia services rendered on other dates within the measurement window (ie, for repeat colonoscopies or other related procedures) may still be captured as related to the episode; hence, the $2 of general anesthesia services captured for the "No Anesthesia" group's episodes, on average.

average costs are not materially different between the 2 groups across the other types of service provided.

DISCUSSION

We have developed an initial measure specification to examine resource use associated with a colonoscopy episode. The measure was developed through a consensus process that included the representation of key clinical stakeholders who are actively involved in colorectal cancer screening and treatment. The measure includes resource use related to the procedure itself, as well as the pertinent resource use both related to preparations in advance of the procedure and related to any complications that may result. When testing the measure in a commercially insured population, we found that the average cost of a colonoscopy episode was just under $1200 and that the predominating contributing elements were the procedure costs ($658 or 55.2%) and outpatient facility costs ($359 or 30.1%).

The work group suspected that the use of general anesthesia might be a major factor in differentiating overall resource use in the colonoscopy episode cost of care measure. We found that approximately one-fourth of colonoscopies done were performed with the use of general anesthesia. The cost of these episodes was $448 (42%) higher than those where anesthesia services were not provided as part of the procedure. Although the use of anesthesia may make patients undergoing colonoscopy more comfortable, currently there are no evidence-based guidelines that indicate colonoscopy should be performed under general anesthesia for most of the population. Additionally, there are no data that suggest the use of general anesthesia is associated with better outcomes. From the perspective of the health care system, the use of general anesthesia for colonoscopy may represent an inefficient use of resources if the costs of the episode are higher with no difference in the rates of complications. One question for future study may be whether or not patients would be willing to pay out of pocket for the additional cost of general anesthesia if they believed that it would increase the comfort of having the procedure done.

As noted earlier, the variability in costs observed in the colonoscopy episode is generally less than the variability we have observed in many of the C3 project's other episodes. One factor contributing to this lack of variation is the relatively short duration of the colonoscopy episode—the episode lasts only 22 days. Another is the relative infrequency of complications. However, there is clearly a meaningful difference in the costs between those episodes that use general anesthesia and those episodes that do not. Additionally, because episode costs are 22% higher than the mean ($1455 vs $1192) at the 75th percentile and 70% higher at the 90th percentile, there may be factors other than use of general anesthesia that are associated with higher episode costs. Therefore, this measure may provide additional actionable information if the costs of colonoscopies rendered by a particular provider or group of providers are significantly higher than those of their peer group. Also, despite the relatively low overall level of variability in this episode, it is important to note that because the volume of these procedures nationwide is so significant, even smaller levels of variability are associated with significant potentially unwarranted health care spending.

Two key strengths of this measure, and the development of such episode-based measures in general through the C3 project, are the transparency of the process through which the measures are developed and the use of input from key stakeholders throughout. By contrast, when considering many of the current episode grouping software available commercially, it is not clear what defines an episode or what resource use is assigned to that episode. One objective of this project was to make it clear to the measures' end users exactly what resources were being counted when calculating each episode's costs. This transparency can ultimately help improve the acceptability of the measure by all stakeholder groups.

As stated earlier, a real strength of the project that affects the ultimate acceptability of the measure is the involvement of key stakeholders. The colonoscopy work group was composed of clinicians nominated by professional societies, health plan representatives, and measurement experts. The fact that the measure was developed through a consensus process involving each of these key stakeholders provides for a measure that is meaningful and balanced from both the provider and health plan perspectives. This may ultimately affect the acceptability of the measures in both the physician and payer communities given that they will have a clear understanding of the measure's development process and that their interests were represented throughout the process.

There are a few limitations with our measure that should be noted. First, we require only a 1-year period in which a patient had not received a colonoscopy for the patient to be included in the measure. The HEDIS measure for colorectal cancer screening uses a 10-year look-back period in accordance with screening recommendations. We are unable to look back that far because of data constraints, noting that most users of these measures would likewise be unable to look back for colon cancer screening over a 10-year period. Therefore, patients included in this measure may be those having a colonoscopy for a reason other than a colorectal cancer screening, as they may have had a screening in the past 10 years. However, this measure is aimed at the resource use associated with the colonoscopy and therefore whether or not a previous colon cancer screening was performed may be of less importance than it is with a colorectal cancer screening quality measure.

As with all episode-based measures that use administrative data, we rely on ICD-9, CPT, and other similar codes to identify related services during the episode's measurement window. Therefore, differences in coding practices or coding errors can affect the resources that are included as part of this measure. Our measure is based on inclusion of resource use from a list of related codes and does not exclude any resource use based on the presence of ICD-9 or CPT codes. Therefore, it is possible that a claim will be included in the resource use for an episode if an eligible diagnosis code shows up in any position on the claim regardless of what the procedure or event is associated with the claim. This situation could result in some unrelated resource use being grouped as related. Similarly, it is possible that some resource use (for example a specific procedure) will not group to the episode in some claims and will group with others because of the diagnosis codes on the claim. We would anticipate that this is generally random variability added to the measure and would not result in any systematic differences in resource use.

The findings presented here are based on resource use and practice patterns in 2007; recent decisions by payers relative to the use of anesthesia may result in different findings if the analysis were repeated on a more recent dataset. The results are also not risk adjusted and describe initial findings used in development of the measure specification. Finally, because the goal of this article was to describe the process used for the development of a colonoscopy resource use measure, provide a description of the measure, and present initial findings from the development phase of the project, findings from this article may change as the measure undergoes further refinement and testing.

SUMMARY

Working with a group of key stakeholders, we have developed an episode-based resource use measure focused on the use of colonoscopy. This measure is intended to identify differences in health care resource use in a short time frame surrounding the colonoscopy. It was a goal of this effort to develop a resource use measure that would provide actionable information for the health care community. Although this measure focuses strictly on resource use, it was the ultimate intent in the development of this measure to pair it with a measure of quality so that both the cost and quality of care can be evaluated together. In our initial testing of the episode, we found the use of general anesthesia with colonoscopy to be associated with higher episode costs. It will be important to continue to evaluate the performance of the episode measure in a variety of datasets and populations. Eventually, when paired with quality measures, it is hoped this measure will provide actionable information for health care payers and providers to more efficiently provide colonoscopy services without compromising quality.

ACKNOWLEDGMENTS

The authors gratefully acknowledge the contribution of the clinical experts on the C3 colon cancer work group: John Allen (American Gastroenterological Association), William Bowman (Moses Cone Health System), Samuel Durso (American Geriatrics Society), C. Daniel Johnson (American College of Radiology), David Kirlin (American Society of Clinical Oncology), Bruce Minsky (American Society for Radiation Oncology), Amita Rastogi (Prometheus), Stephen Scott (American Academy of Family

Physicians), Anthony Senagore (American Society of Colon and Rectal Surgeons), and V.O. Speights (College of American Pathologists). The authors also wish to acknowledge the contributions of other members of the C3 Project staff: Robin Wagner (ABMS REF), Larry Manheim (Northwestern University), Kevin Stroupe (Northwestern University), Katie Harrell (ABMS REF), and James Unti (Consultant).

REFERENCES

1. Fisher E, Goodman D, Skinner J, et al. Health care spending, quality, and outcomes: more isn't always better. Dartmouth Atlas Project 2009. Available at: http://www.dartmouthatlas.org/atlases/Spending_Brief_022709.pdf. Accessed January 11, 2010.
2. Wennberg JE. Dealing with medical practice variations: a proposal for action. Health Aff 1984;3:6–32.
3. Fuchs V, McClellan M, Skinner J. Area differences in utilization of medical care and mortality among US elderly. Cambridge (MA): National Bureau of Economic Research (NBER) Working Paper No. 8628, December 2001.
4. Brownlee S. Overtreated: why too much medicine is making us sicker and poorer. New York: Bloomsbury USA; 2007.
5. Centers for Disease Control and Prevention. Colorectal cancer statistics. Available at: http://www.cdc.gov/cancer/colorectal/statistics/index.htm. Accessed January 11, 2010.
6. Alliance AQ. Candidate list of conditions for cost of care measurement. Available at: http://www.aqaalliance.org/files/CandidateListofConditionsforCostofCare MeasurementApproved.pdf. Accessed January 11, 2010.
7. Baxter NN, Goldwasser MA, Paszat LF, et al. Association of colonoscopy and death from colorectal cancer. Ann Intern Med 2009;150:1–8.
8. Ransohoff DF. Have we oversold colonoscopy? Gastroenterology 2005;129:1815.
9. National Cancer Institute. Fact sheet: colorectal screening. Available at: http://www.cancer.gov/cancertopics/factsheet/Detection/colorectal-screening. Accessed January 11, 2010.
10. Rex D, Johnson D, Anderson J, et al. American College of Gastroenterology guidelines for colorectal cancer screening 2009. Am J Gastroenterol 2009;104:139–50.
11. Adams K, Corrigan J, editors. Priority areas for national action: transforming health care quality. Institute of Medicine. Washington, DC: National Academies Press; 2003. p. 117–25.
12. Meissner HI, Breen N, Klabunde CN, et al. Patterns of colorectal cancer screening uptake among men and women in the United States. Cancer Epidemiol Biomarkers Prev 2006;15:389–94.
13. Harewood GC, Lieberman DA. Colonoscopy practice patterns since introduction of Medicare coverage for average-risk screening. Clin Gastroenterol Hepatol. 2004;2:72–7.
14. Leung FW, Aharonian HS, Guth PH, et al. Unsedated colonoscopy: time to revisit this option? J Fam Pract 2008;57:E1–4.
15. Witt TN, Enns R. The difficult colonoscopy. Can J Gastroenterol 2007;21:487–90.
16. Arrowsmith JB, Gerstman BB, Fleischer DE, et al. Results from the American Society for Gastrointestinal Endoscopy/US Food and Drug Administration collaborative study on complication rates and drug use during gastrointestinal endoscopy. Gastrointest Endosc 1991;37:421–7.
17. Sharma VK, Nguyen C, Crowell MD, et al. A national study of cardiopulmonary unplanned events after GI endoscopy. Gastrointest Endosc 2007;66:27–34.

18. Pham HH, Schrag D, O'Malley AS, et al. Care patterns in Medicare and their implications for pay for performance. N Engl J Med 2007;356:1130–9.

19. Available at: http://www.ingenix.com/ThoughtLeadership/ETG/ETGpapers/. Accessed January 11, 2010.

20. Available at: http://thomsonreuters.com/content/healthcare/white_papers/medical_episode_grouper_transpar. Accessed January 11, 2010

21. Lake T, Colby M, Peterson S. Health plans use of physician resource use and quality measures. Available at: http://www.medpac.gov/documents/6355%20MedPAC%20Final%20Report%20with%20Appendices%201-24-08.pdf. Accessed January 29, 2010.

22. Warren JL, Klabunde CN, Mariotto AB, et al. Adverse events after outpatient colonoscopy in the Medicare population. Ann Intern Med 2009;150:849–57.

Cost-effectiveness of Colonoscopy

Ann G. Zauber, PhD

KEYWORDS

- Colonoscopy • Colorectal cancer screening
- Cost-effectiveness analysis
- Comparative effectiveness research • Efficient frontier

Colonoscopy was first recommended as a primary screening test for colorectal cancer (CRC) in the 1997 Guidelines of the GI Consortium,[1] which provided a menu of CRC screening options. This recommendation was based on the ability to use colonoscopy to see and remove the precursor lesion within the same colonoscopic examination across the entire colon and rectum. Clinical evidence for using colonoscopy as a screening tool[1] was based on 3 lines of evidence: (1) the mortality reduction achieved by colonoscopies performed for positive fecal occult blood tests (FOBT) in randomized controlled trials of the Hemoccult II guaiac-based FOBT[2–4]; (2) the mortality reduction of rigid sigmoidoscopy in case-control studies[5,6]; and (3) the reduction in CRC incidence in the National Polyp Study with colonoscopic polypectomy.[7] Colonoscopy is now recommended as one of the primary CRC screening tests by (1) the United States Preventive Services Task Force (USPSTF),[8] (2) the combined organizations of the American Cancer Society, US Multi-Society Task Force on Colorectal Cancer representing multiple gastroenterology societies, and the American College of Radiology[9] (ACS-MSTF-ACR), and (3) the American College of Gastroenterology (ACG).[10] Each organization presents colonoscopy as one option for CRC screening, with the ACG citing colonoscopy as the primary CRC screening test.[10]

This article compares the recommendations for CRC screening tests by the different organizations. In addition a cost-effectiveness analysis (CEA) of these strategies that we reported to the Center for Medicare and Medicaid Services (CMS)[11] and a recent analysis of the different strategies relative to computed tomographic colonography (CTC) are reviewed.[12] This review of the cost-effectiveness results of the different strategies provides further context to understand the risks and benefits of the recommended strategies in practice.

Dr Zauber is supported in part by Cancer Intervention and Surveillance Modeling Network grants from the National Cancer Institute: (U01-CA-097426 and U01-CA-115953).
Conflict of interest: none.
Department of Epidemiology and Biostatistics, Memorial Sloan-Kettering Cancer Center, 307 East 63rd Street, Room 357, New York, NY 10065, USA
E-mail address: zaubera@mskcc.org

Gastrointest Endoscopy Clin N Am 20 (2010) 751–770
doi:10.1016/j.giec.2010.07.008
1052-5157/10/$ – see front matter © 2010 Elsevier Inc. All rights reserved.

RECOMMENDATIONS FOR CRC SCREENING FROM 3 ORGANIZATIONS

The recommendations from the 3 organizations for CRC screening tests are presented in **Table 1**. Although similar evidence was reviewed by these 3 groups, there were differences in the test strategies recommended. The USPSTF and the ACS-MSTF-ACR present a menu of options, whereas the ACG presents preferred strategy options. The USPSTF formally evaluated risks and benefits of screening for the average risk patient and concluded that there was insufficient evidence at this time to recommend CTC or stool DNA testing for the general population.[8] Both of these tests were included in the ACS-MSTF-ACR and ACG recommendations, but with the caveat that the interval of screening with the stool DNA test is not yet established. Furthermore, there has been discussion of the minimum size of polyp detected by CTC for referral to colonoscopy. (The ACS-MSTF-ACR did recommend that all CTC polyps of 6 mm or larger would be referred for colonoscopy.)

Tests recommended in common by all 3 groups are colonoscopy and the more sensitive FOBTs (fecal immunochemical tests [FIT] [preferred] or guaiac Hemoccult SENSA, Beckman Coulter, Brea, CA, USA). Flexible sigmoidoscopy every 5 years in conjunction with a sensitive FOBT (SENSA or FIT) every 2 to 3 years is recommended by the USPSTF, whereas flexible sigmoidoscopy alone or Hemoccult II alone is not recommended. However, the ACS-MSTF-ACR include flexible sigmoidoscopy and barium enema as individual tests in their recommendations.

Table 1
Comparison of CRC screening guidelines from the USPSTF, the ACS-MSTF-ACR, and the ACG

	USPSTF[8]	ACS-MSTF-ACR[9]	ACG[10]
Age to Begin, Stop			
Age to start screening	50 years	50 years	50 years (begin age 45 years for African Americans)
Age to stop screening	75 years	None stated	None stated
Age to stop surveillance for adenoma and CRC subjects	None	None	None
Recommended Tests			
Hemoccult II (annual)	No	No	No
Hemoccult SENSA (annual)	Yes	Yes	Yes
FIT (annual)	Yes	Yes	Yes (first preferred alternative test if subject refuses colonoscopy)
Flexible sigmoidoscopy (every 5 years)	No	Yes	Alternative test if colonoscopy refusal
Flexible sigmoidoscopy (every 5 years) with sensitive FOBT (every 2–3 y)	Yes	Not stated	Not stated
Colonoscopy (every 10 y)	Yes	Yes	Yes (as first choice)
CTC (every 5 y for ≥6 mm polyps)	No (insufficient evidence)	Yes	Yes (alternative test if subject refuses colonoscopy)
Stool DNA (interval not set)	No (insufficient evidence)	Yes	Yes (alternative test if subject refuses colonoscopy)
Double-contrast barium enema	No	Yes	No

The ACS-MSTF-ACR also classify the screening tests as (1) those that can prevent cancer through early detection of adenomas as well as detect CRC (recommended tests of colonoscopy every 10 years, flexible sigmoidoscopy every 5 years, CTC every 5 years, and double-contrast barium enema every 5 years) and (2) those that can primarily detect CRC early (recommended tests of annual guaiac-based FOBT with high test sensitivity for cancer, annual FIT with high test sensitivity for cancer, or stool DNA test with high sensitivity for cancer, interval uncertain). High test sensitivity for cancer was defined as 50% or greater for testing at one point in time. Furthermore, the ACS-MSTF-ACR guidelines state that the primary goal of screening should be to prevent CRC.

The ACG recommends that clinicians have access to a preferred strategy as an alternative to a menu of options. The ACG recommends the cancer prevention test of colonscopy as the first option, and then the FIT as the first alternative. Additional alternative tests include flexible sigmoidoscopy every 5 to 10 years, CTC every 5 years, Hemoccult SENSA annually, and stool DNA testing every 3 years. The ACG also grades its recommendations according to the amount of evidence supporting the recommendation and the benefit versus risk of the strategies. Colonoscopy, FIT, annual Hemoccult SENSA, and FIT have recommendation level 1B, which denotes strong recommendation with moderate quality evidence.

Thus, recommendations from different organizations vary because the rationale behind their recommendations differs.

COMPARATIVE EFFECTIVENESS RESEARCH TO COMPARE CRC SCREENING TESTS

In comparing screening tests, both the risk and benefits of screening for each particular test are considered. Risks are commonly represented by the costs and benefits by life-years gained (LYG). Incidence or mortality reduction obtained with screening can also be used to represent benefits. Comparative effectiveness research is the conduct and synthesis of research comparing the benefits and harms of various interventions and strategies for preventing, diagnosing, treating, and monitoring health conditions in real-world settings. The purpose is to improve health outcomes by developing and disseminating evidence-based information to patients, clinicians, and other decision makers about which interventions are most effective for which patients under specific circumstances.[13]

In this article the cost-effectiveness of the recommended CRC screening tests is discussed, and in particular the relationship of colonoscopy to other tests for screening in the average risk population. FOBT (Hemoccult II, Hemoccult SENSA, FIT), flexible sigmoidoscopy alone with and without biopsy, flexible sigmoidoscopy with annual Hemoccult II and with annual Hemoccult SENSA, and colonoscopy are included. Because the CMS has not approved either CTC or stool DNA testing for CRC screening, there are no Medicare reimbursement rates for these tests. Our previous results of CEAs that we carried out for CMS in relationship to CT colonoscopy to assess a potential reimbursement level are summarized.[11,12] Stool DNA testing is not included in this CEA. The capsule endoscopy is not discussed[14] because there is insufficient evidence for effectiveness[15] and it has not been included in any screening guidelines to date.

CEA of CRC screening tests has been conducted with varying cost structures and assumptions and has produced varying conclusions. In 2002, Pignone and colleagues[16] provided a systematic review of CEA for CRC screening in the United States from 5 models[17–21] and reported that the strategies of colonoscopy, sigmoidoscopy with or without FOBT (Hemoccult II), and FOBT alone all provided screening strategies that were less than $50,000 per life-year gained compared with no screening. However, no screening test strategy was consistently the most effective CRC strategy when they were compared with each other across the 5 models. To improve this situation the Institute of Medicine (IOM) convened a conference in 2004 to assess CRC screening CEAs. Representatives from each of the 5 models originally reviewed by Pignone and colleagues[22] were asked to present at the January 2004 IOM conference and provide costs and LYG for 5 screening strategies (colonoscopy, sigmoidoscopy, sigmoidoscopy plus FOBT, FOBT alone, and a test similar to barium enema) under their original assumptions and again with standardized input assumptions concerning test characteristics, adherence to screening (100%), follow-up, and surveillance as well as for test costs and treatment costs.[23] With standardized inputs, the models still varied in the absolute levels of costs and LYG, but the relative ordering of strategies with respect to cost-effectiveness results was comparable. Given a willingness to pay of $20,000 or $50,000 per life-year saved, the preferred strategy was annual FOBT. However, sigmoidoscopy plus annual FOBT was the preferred strategy in 4 of 5 models, for a willingness to pay of $100,000 per life-year saved.

MICROSIMULATION MODELING TO INFORM HEALTH POLICY

Although randomized controlled trials are the preferred method for establishing effectiveness of (screening) interventions, they are expensive, require long follow-up, and can include only a few comparison tests. Therefore, well-validated microsimulation models may be used to estimate the required resources and expected benefits from different screening policies and inform decision making. There are 3 CRC microsimulation models in the National Cancer Institute's Cancer Intervention and Surveillance Modeling Network (CISNET). The models are based on clinical incidence data before the introduction of screening (1975–1979) Surveillance, Epidemiology, and End Results [SEER] data[24] and on the size distribution of adenomas in colonoscopy and autopsy studies.[25–34] They have been validated against the long-term reductions in incidence and mortality of CRC with annual FOBT reported in the randomized controlled trial of the Minnesota Colon Cancer Control Study[2,35,36] and show good concordance with the trial results. Transparency of the models is provided through standardized profiles of the structure of each model, and underlying model parameters and assumptions are available at http://cisnet.cancer.gov/profiles/.

In this article, the results from one of the CISNET models (MISCAN: Microsimulation Screening Analysis, from Erasmus University Medical Center and Memorial–Sloan-Kettering Cancer Center) are used to provide CEA of the screening tests recommended by the 3 guideline groups. The results are from the CEA for CMS on CTC[11] and a recent analysis of the different strategies relative to CTC.[12] The primary analysis for this work was for a cohort of those 65 years of age. In this article the results of the secondary analysis for a cohort of those 50 years of age are used.

The MISCAN model simulates the life histories of a large population from birth to death in 2 situations: the natural history of the adenoma-carcinoma sequence and the effect of the screening intervention to detect and remove adenomas or CRC. As each simulated individual ages, there is a chance that an adenomatous polyp (a benign precursor lesion that may lead to CRC) may develop. One or more adenomas can occur in any individual and each can develop into preclinical CRC. The risk of developing an adenoma may depend on age, sex, genetic, and other propensity factors. Adenomas can grow and eventually some of them can become malignant, transforming to stage I preclinical cancer. A preclinical cancer (ie, not detected) has a chance of progressing through the stages (from stages I to IV) and may be detected by symptoms at any stage. The authors assume that adenomas are asymptomatic and can be detected only by a screening test (**Fig. 1**).

The effectiveness of each screening test is modeled through the ability of each test to detect lesions (ie, adenomas, preclinical cancer). Once screening is introduced, a simulated person who has developed an underlying adenoma or preclinical cancer has a chance of having it detected during a screening episode depending on the sensitivity of the test for that lesion. For screened persons without an underlying lesion we apply the false-positive rate (1–specificity) to determine whether or not that person will undergo an unnecessary follow-up examination. Hyperplastic polyps are not modeled explicitly but are reflected in the specificity of the test. Furthermore, a percentage of individuals with false-negative test results (ie, adenoma or preclinical cancer present but not detected) are referred to colonoscopy because of the detection of a hyperplastic polyp.

STUDY POPULATION

We used the natural history model to estimate the distribution of underlying disease in terms of the presence, location, size, and type (adenoma vs preclinical cancer) of lesions. We conducted an analysis of the effect of different screening strategies among a cohort of 50-year-old individuals in the US population in 2005 who have never been screened as our base case.

TEST STRATEGIES

A test strategy includes the initial screening test as well as follow-up diagnosis of a positive test, diagnosis, and treatment of CRC and recurrent cancer, surveillance

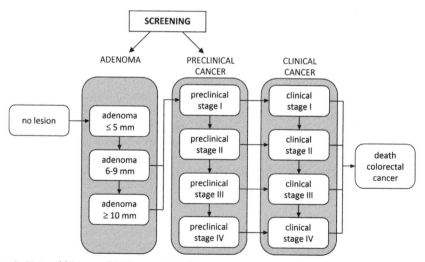

Fig. 1. Natural history of CRC as modeled by MISCAN model. Screening provides the opportunity to intervene in the natural history of the adenoma-carcinoma sequence. Screening can either remove a precancerous lesion (ie, adenoma), thus moving a person to the "no lesion" state, or provide early cancer detection, which makes an undiagnosed cancer clinically detected at a potentially earlier stage of disease when it is more amenable to treatment.

colonoscopy for those with adenomas, and treatment of any complications from screening. We compared the strategies of screening with FOBT every year, flexible sigmoidoscopy every 5 years, combinations of annual FOBT and sigmoidoscopy (every 5 years), and colonoscopy every 10 years. Although double-contrast barium enema was included in the 2002 screening recommendations for the USPSTF,[37] it was not included in the 2008 USPSTF recommendations and is not considered in this analysis. We evaluated 3 FOBTs (Hemoccult II, Hemoccult SENSA, and FIT) and 2 strategies for sigmoidoscopy (with and without biopsy and also with and without FOBT), and 2 representations for CTC for a total of 14 screening strategies plus no screening.

We assumed that all individuals begin CRC screening at age 50 years as recommended by all 3 screening guidelines and end at age 80 years. A patient with a positive screening test is referred for colonoscopy. If adenomas are detected on colonoscopy then the individual begins surveillance with colonoscopy per the 2006 guidelines from the joint publication of the US Multi-Society Task Force and the American Cancer Society.[9,38] The cohort was followed for their lifetimes to a maximum of age 100 years. The LYG per strategy were derived relative to no screening.

CRC SCREENING TEST CHARACTERISTICS

The sensitivity and specificity of the FOBTs were based on a literature review[39,40] and were consistent with those from the 2008 review of the evidence on CRC screening tests for the USPSTF.[41] There are multiple FITs with varying cut points for positivity, number of slides, number of days tested, and preparations reported in the literature.[39] Consequently FIT sensitivity and specificity criteria vary widely. The OC-Sensor FIT has recently been used in clinical trials in Holland[42] and Northern California at Kaiser Permanente (TR Levin, personal communication, 2010). Sensitivities for colonoscopy were based on a meta-analysis[43]; we assumed the same sensitivities for sigmoidoscopy within the reach of the endoscope. We assumed that 5% of subjects have more than one colonoscopy to visualize the entire colon and that the cecum is ultimately reached in 98% of subjects. For sigmoidoscopy, we assumed that 80% of examinations reach the junction of the sigmoid and descending colon and 40% reach the beginning of the splenic flexure.[44,45] The test characteristics were consistent with the evidence review used in the USPSTF recommendations.[41] The test characteristics for CTC were based on 2 clinical trials: Department of Defense (DoD)[46] and the National CT Colonography Trial (ACRIN 6664).[47]

Table 2 contains an overview of test characteristics used in our analyses. Test parameters are given by person for the fecal tests and by lesion for colonoscopy, flexible sigmoidoscopy, and CTC. The sensitivities stated in **Table 2** are based on sensitivities of the test at one point in time. However, the LYG and the costs for each test strategy are based on repeated screening.

COSTS

Cost reimbursements for the components of screening vary by type of insurance plans, and copayments. In this article we present as an example the derivation of costs of a screening strategy based on Medicare reimbursement (without copayments) for each of the recommended screening tests and use these costs in conjunction with the MISCAN microsimulation model for the LYG with screening for each test. We recognize that costs vary in practice but use Medicare reimbursement without copayments as one standardized measure for costs.

Table 2
Test characteristics for CRC screening tests

| Test | Sensitivity[a] by Adenoma Size or CRC (%) | | | | Specificity (%) |
	≤5 mm	6–9 mm	≥10 mm	CRC	
Per Person					
Hemoccult II	2.0	5.0	12.0	40.0	98.0
Hemoccult SENSA	7.5	12.4	23.9	70.0	92.5
FIT	5.0	10.1	22.0	70.0	95.0
Per Lesion and Within Reach					
Sigmoidoscopy (within reach)[b]	75.0	85.0	95.0	95.0	92.0[c]
Colonoscopy	75.0	85.0	95.0	95.0	90.0[c]
CTC DoD 3D 6 mm	–	83.6[d]	92.2	92.2[e]	79.6[f]
CTC ACRIN NCTC 2D/3D 6 mm	–	57.0[d]	84.0	84.0[e]	88.0[f]

Abbreviations: DoD, Department of Defense study[46,79]; NCTC, National CT Colonography Trial[47]; –, indicates sensitivity is not provided because size is smaller than the colonoscopy referral threshold of 6 mm; 2D, two-dimensional; 3D, three-dimensional.

[a] Sensitivity is provided per individual for stool-based tests and per lesion for endoscopy and CTC tests.

[b] Test characteristics for sigmoidoscopy apply only to lesions in the distal colon and rectum.

[c] The lack of specificity with sigmoidoscopy and colonoscopy reflects the detection of nonadenomatous lesions. With sigmoidoscopy, the presence of nonadenomatous lesions induces biopsy costs (in the case of sigmoidoscopy with biopsy) or results in referral for colonoscopy (in the case of sigmoidoscopy without biopsy). With colonoscopy, nonadenomatous lesions are removed and therefore induce polypectomy and biopsy costs.

[d] Sensitivity for CTC for adenomas 6 to 9 mm was mathematically derived from published tables.

[e] Sensitivity for CRC was assumed to be the same as for adenomas of size 10 mm or larger because of the small number of CRCs detected in the DoD and NCTC studies.

[f] The lack of specificity with CTC reflects the detection of nonadenomatous polyps, artifacts, and adenomas smaller than the colonoscopy referral threshold of 6 mm.

Payer's Perspective

The base case CEA was from the payer's (CMS) perspective with costs stated as those that Medicare pays and based on Medicare payments of 2007 for procedures and tests associated with CRC screening, complications of screening, and treatment.[48] These payments reflect approximately 80% of the allowable charge, including the facility charges (as applicable) and physician services charges. (Thus the beneficiary's copay is not reflected in the analysis.) We also conducted an analysis from a modified societal perspective by including direct costs borne by beneficiaries as well as estimated patient time costs, but excluding costs caused by lost productivity caused by early death or disability.

The screening test costs are provided in **Table 3**. Screening-related costs are based on the set of current procedural terminology (CPT) codes relevant to CRC screening in conjunction with the points of service for the procedures: (1) in the Ambulatory Surgery Center (ASC) setting, we include the Medicare ASC facility payment and the payment for physician professional services; (2) in the Outpatient Prospective Payment System (OPPS) setting, we include the Medicare OPPS facility payment and the payment for physician services; and (3) in the office setting, we include the payment to the physician that covers both the professional services and the facility costs of the physician's office. The total costs per CPT code are weighted by the frequencies for points of service. Then the total costs per screening procedure are based on the total costs

Table 3
Screening test costs based on CMS payment (2007 US dollars)

Screening Test	CMS Cost ($)[a]	Modified Societal Cost ($)[b]
Guaiac Hemoccult (II or SENSA)	4.54	21.54
FIT	22.22	39.22
Flexible sigmoidoscopy	160.78	270.30
Flexible sigmoidoscopy with biopsy	348.19	497.37
Colonoscopy without polypectomy[c]	497.59	794.94
Colonoscopy with polypectomy or biopsy[c]	648.52	979.28
CTC[a,d]	488.29	643.64

[a] CMS cost represents approximately 80% of the allowable charge in 2007 US dollars.
[b] Modified societal costs include beneficiary costs (copayments) and time costs in addition to the payer costs.
[c] Base case cost for colonoscopy does not include additional anesthesia costs. A secondary sensitivity analysis in the CMS report considers an additional $74 cost added to colonoscopy for anesthesia in 29% and 100% of colonoscopies.[11]
[d] Based on CMS payment for CT of the abdomen (CPT 74150), CT of the pelvis (CPT 72192), and image processing on an independent workstation (CPT 76377). No screening cost for CMS has been established.

per CPT code that are part of the procedure and weighted by the frequencies of the CPT codes. Payments for a procedure across these settings are represented as an average of the 3 settings weighted by the frequency of which each setting is used for the procedure in 2007. We do not include the cost of a separate office visit for any of the screening strategies as we assume that all recommendations or arrangements for screening would already be associated with a previously scheduled office visit. Payer cost for Hemoccult II, Hemoccult SENSA, and fecal immunochemical testing does not include additional charges for points of service because these costs are related only to the clinical laboratory fee schedule (http://www.cms.hhs.gov/ClinicalLabFeeSched/).

Given that CTC has not been approved for screening in the Medicare population, there is no national CMS payment rate for a screening CTC. Accordingly, we used as a proxy the national average CMS payment for an abdominal CT without contrast (CPT code 74150), a pelvic CT without contrast (CPT code 72192), and image processing on an independent workstation (CPT 76377). This base case cost estimate of CTC of $488.29 does not include costs for further radiological evaluations for extracolonic findings.[11]

Screening Test Costs

The costs for colonoscopy without polypectomy were based on CPT codes 45378 (diagnostic colonoscopy), G0105 (colon screen in high risk individuals), and G0121 (colon cancer screening for nonhigh-risk individual). Costs for colonoscopy with polypectomy or biopsy were composed of codes 45380 (colonoscopy and biopsy), 45381 (colonoscopy, submucous injection), 45382 (colonoscopy/control bleeding), 45383 (lesion removal colonoscopy-fulguration), 45384 (lesion removal colonoscopy-hot biopsy), and 45385 (lesion removal colonoscopy-snare polypectomy).

We assumed that polypectomy was not performed with flexible sigmoidoscopy screening. However, we distinguished flexible sigmoidoscopy with and without biopsy. For flexible sigmoidoscopy without biopsy we used CPT codes 45330 (diagnostic sigmoidoscopy) and G0104 (CA screen; flexi sigmoidoscope). Flexible sigmoidoscopy with biopsy was based on CPT code 45331 (sigmoidoscopy and biopsy).

Polyp Removal and Pathology Review

For the procedures with polypectomy or biopsy we included a pathology charge (CPT code 88305). The Medicare payment rates per jar were $82.40 for the physician fee schedule for office and ASC settings, and $51.59 for the OPPS setting. We assumed that all biopsies and removed polyps are reviewed by a pathologist and that a separate jar is submitted for each of 4 colon segments so the resection area can be identified should surgery be necessary. Data from the National Colonoscopy Study were used to provide the estimate of 1.38 as the average number of jars per patient with polyps (hyperplastic, other polyps, and adenomas) (Ann Zauber, PhD, personal communication). Consequently, we multiplied the pathology fee by 1.38 to obtain the average pathology cost associated with colonoscopy with polypectomy.

Multiple polyps requiring the same type of polypectomy removal within a single colonoscopy do not add an incremental cost to the procedure. However, if different types of polypectomy are required in removing multiple polyps then CMS reimburses 100% for the most expensive procedure and 50% of the facility cost for the second procedure. As a simplifying assumption we use the weights of procedures by CPT type and do not consider different fees for different combinations of endoscopy CPT codes for polyp removal.

Anesthesia Cost for Colonoscopy

For the base case the cost of moderate sedation was included in the cost of colonoscopy, assuming that it is not administered by an anesthesiologist. Some anesthesia costs such as monitored anesthesia care (MAC) provided by an anesthesia professional are currently being reimbursed in addition to the colonoscopy procedure. The additional CMS payment for the anesthesia was $74, based on an average cost for the CPT code 00810 in 2007 for MAC for lower endoscopy procedures.

Complications of Screening

There are essentially no complications from the stool-based screening tests (Hemoccult II, Hemoccult SENSA, or FIT). However, patients undergoing colonoscopy and, to a lesser extent, flexible sigmoidoscopy and CTC are at risk of experiencing complications from the procedures. Because individuals with a positive FOBT, sigmoidoscopy, or CTC are referred for a follow-up colonoscopy, the complications and the associated costs are relevant and accounted for in all of the screening strategies.

The major complications of colonoscopy are perforations, which can occur with or without polypectomy, serosal burns, bleeds requiring transfusion, and bleeds not requiring transfusion.[49–53] The costs of complications were based on the relevant diagnosis-related group codes (**Table 4**). Risks of complications reported in organized screening programs[50,51,54] are lower than those reported for general practice colonoscopies[49,55] and increase with increasing age.[53,56] Overall risks of complications of colonoscopy have declined. Our estimates for colonoscopy risks are similar to a population-based study in Canada[57] with rates of 1.64 per 1000 for bleeding and 0.85 per 1000 for perforation. They are also consistent with the evidence review by Whitlock and colleagues,[41] who stated that complication rates could not be derived for colonoscopies with and without polypectomy because of reporting limitations.

Table 4
Summary of risks of complications and costs (2007 US dollars)

Complication	Rate Per 1000	CMS Cost ($)	Modified Societal Cost ($)
With Colonoscopy			
Perforation	0.7	12,446	12,712
Serosal burn	0.3	5208	5474
Bleed with transfusion	0.4	5208	5474
Bleed without transfusion	1.1	320	586
With Flexible Sigmoidoscopy			
Perforation	0.02	12,446	12,712
With CTC			
Perforation	0.0456	12,446	12,712

Costs for CRC Treatment

The net costs of CRC treatment are derived from a comparison of costs for CRC cases relative to those of matched controls in the SEER-Medicare files for the years 1998 to 2003[58] and vary by phase of care (**Table 5**). The initial phase is the first 12 months following diagnosis, the last-year-of-life phase is the final 12 months of life, and the continuing phase is the months between initial and last year. This methodology was used previously by Brown and colleagues[59] to assess net costs of cancer treatment.

CEA

To conduct a CEA we use the MISCAN microsimulation model to calculate the lifetime costs and life expectancy for a previously unscreened cohort of 50-year-old individuals residing in the United States under different CRC screening strategies. CEA

Table 5
Net payments for CRC care during 1998 to 2003 (in 2007 US dollars)[a]

American Joint Committee on Cancer Stage	Initial Phase	Continuing Phase	Last Year of Life	
			Died of CRC	Died of Other Causes
Direct Medical Costs				
I	25,487	2028	45,689	11,257
II	35,173	1890	45,560	9846
III	42,885	2702	48,006	13,026
IV	56,000	8375	64,428	34,975
Modified Societal Costs				
I	32,720	2719	56,640	17,408
II	43,752	2561	56,417	15,740
III	53,003	3573	59,481	19,413
IV	68,853	10,743	78,227	44,384

[a] The initial phase of care is the first 12 months following diagnosis, the last-year-of-life phase is the final 12 months of life, and the continuing phase is all the months between the initial and last-year-of-life phases. Cancer-related costs in the continuing phase of care are an annual estimate.

does not select which strategy is economically preferred overall, but only which strategy is the most effective, in terms of life-years saved, for a given level of desired (or possible) expenditure.[60]

The first consideration in a CEA is whether a strategy is effective as represented by the LYG with screening without regard for the relative costs of the strategies (**Table 6**). We use an illustration from our analysis for the CMS for CTC[11] to show that the LYG (per 1000) with screening (ie, effectiveness) are lowest for the strategies of annual Hemoccult II only (207 per 1000 screened) and flexible sigmoidoscopy only every 5 years (214 and 222 per 1000 screened) but higher and at approximately the same level of effectiveness for the strategies of sensitive FOBTs with or without flexible sigmoidoscopy every 5 years (238–251 LYG) and colonoscopy every 10 years (243 LYG) under the assumption of 100% adherence for all aspects of testing and follow-up. CTC has a range of 231 to 241 LYG, which is close to the range of the sensitive FOBTs without flexible sigmoidoscopy (238–240 LYG).

The next step in a CEA is assessing the ratio of risks (generally in costs) to benefits (in LYG) with screening. CEA generally discounts its costs by 3% annually to account for the up-front costs of screening, although the benefits arise in the future. Given that

Table 6
CEA for 14 CRC screening strategies considered by one or more of the 3 guideline organizations: LYG, discounted and net costs, ACER, and ICER

| Strategy[a] | LYG | MISCAN Model for LYG and Strategy Costs Per 1000 Screened | | | | |
		Discounted Costs ($)	Net Discounted Costs ($)	Discounted LYG	ACER ($/LYG)	ICER ($/LYG)
No screening	0	2,320,612	0	0.0		–
HII	207	2,369,426	48,814	85.3	572	572
HS	240	2,615,292	294,680	100.2	2941	16,605
FIT	238	2,688,092	367,480	99.7	3686	Dominated
SIGB	222	2,725,559	404,947	89.2	4540	Dominated
SIG	214	2,759,328	438,716	92.2	4758	Dominated
HII + SIGB	246	2,760,602	439,990	103.0	4272	Dominated
HII + SIG	246	2,823,342	502,730	102.9	4886	Dominated
HS + SIGB	248	2,952,372	631,760	104.8	6028	73,336
HS + SIG	249	2,933,686	613,074	104.4	5872	Dominated
FIT + SIGB	250	3,151,945	831,333	105.6	7872	272,160
FIT + SIG	251	3,058,485	737,873	105.0	7027	Dominated
COL	243	3,011,165	690,553	101.8	6783	Dominated
CTC DoD	241	3,685,253	1,364,641	100.6	13,565	Dominated
CTC ACRIN	231	3,751,074	1,430,462	96.1	14,885	Dominated

The strategies in bold type represent the acceptable strategies with respect to LYG and willingness to pay.

Abbreviations: ACER, average cost-effectiveness ratio compared with no screening; COL, colonoscopy; FIT, immunochemical FOBT; HII, Hemoccult II; HS, Hemoccult SENSA; ICER, incremental cost-effectiveness ratio; LYG, life-years gained versus no screening; SIG, sigmoidoscopy without biopsy; SIGB, sigmoidoscopy with biopsy; – indicates default strategy (ie, the least costly and least effective nondominated strategy).

[a] The 2 CTC strategies are not competing options. They are shown here together for comparison purposes only. The ICERs are assessed separately using each CTC strategy in turn.

costs are typically discounted (3%) the LYG are also discounted by 3% in analyses comparing costs and LYG. This discounting reflects the general societal preference to have a dollar in the present rather than in the future.

Cost-effectiveness ratios (CERs) are derived as average or incremental (marginal) measures.[61] An average CER (ACER) is derived without regard to other screening alternatives. It is the discounted cost of the strategy relative to no screening divided by the LYG with screening and shows whether the net benefits of the strategy are a good value for the resources required among individuals who would not be screened at all without the availability of that strategy (see **Table 6**). All the screening options considered have an ACER less than $15,000, which is lower than the commonly accepted level of $50,000 per life-year saved as an acceptable intervention. The strategies, excluding CTC, all had ACERs even less than $8000 per life-year gained.

An incremental analysis is recommended by the Panel on Cost-Effectiveness in Health and Medicine[62] for competing strategies, and shows whether the net benefits of a strategy are a good value for the resources required compared with the other currently available CRC screening strategies; this is the preferred approach in comparative effectiveness research. We conducted an incremental CEA from the perspective of CMS and discounted future costs and life-years 3% annually for our report to CMS on CTC. We did not use quality-adjusted LYG because we did not have good measures on the effects of screening on quality of life, particularly as quality relates to the anxiety of waiting for the results of the screening tests.

The discounted LYG (on the y-axis) plotted against the discounted costs (on the x-axis) for each strategy provide descriptive and quantitative measures of the comparisons of risk with benefit (**Fig. 2**). The higher the point, the more effective the screening strategy.[60] As for the undiscounted analysis, all strategies except Hemoccult II and sigmoidoscopy alone have high LYG. The more to the left, the lower is the cost. The more to the right, the more expensive is the screening strategy. The strategies toward

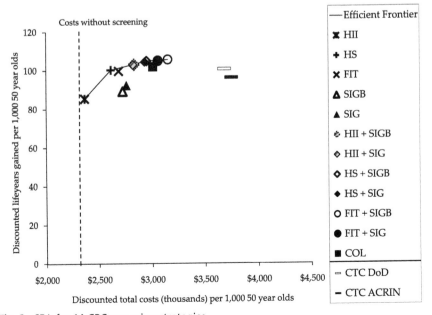

Fig. 2. CEA for 14 CRC screening strategies.

the upper left-hand corner are those with the higher LYG relative to lower costs per LYG. Costs for strategies that include endoscopy are more expensive than those using FOBTs only. Cost is $3,011,165 per 1000 screened for colonoscopy and $3,151,945 for flexible sigmoidoscopy plus FIT. The Hemoccult II strategy is the lowest cost at $2,369,426 per 1000 screened and is almost cost saving compared with the cost of not screening at all of $2,320,612. The highest cost strategy is CTC ($3,685,253–$3,751,074).

For a quantitative comparison of LYG per cost for multiple strategies, we ranked the screening strategies by increasing effectiveness (ie, discounted number of LYG compared with no screening) from annual Hemoccult II with the lowest life-years saved (85.3 per 1000 screened) to flexible sigmoidoscopy with biopsy every 5 years plus annual FIT (105.6 per 1000 screened) and compared their life-years saved relative to the cost of the strategy. In **Fig. 2** for the plot of LYG versus costs, the black line links the strategies with the most LYG relative to a given level of costs and is called the efficient frontier. These strategies represent the set of efficient options and include Hemoccult II, Hemoccult SENSA, flexible sigmoidoscopy with biopsy and annual Hemoccult SENSA, and flexible sigmoidoscopy with biopsy and annual FIT. Strategies that are more costly and less effective (fewer LYG) than another strategy are below the efficient frontier and are considered dominated by the more efficient strategies. These dominated strategies include FIT, sigmoidoscopy alone, 4 of the flexible sigmoidoscopy and FOBT combinations, colonoscopy, and CTC. However, the only strategies relatively far off the efficient frontier (ie, a dominated strategy) are flexible sigmoidoscopy alone and CTC. The other dominated strategies (including colonoscopy) are close to that of the efficient frontier and could be considered in the set of acceptable cost-effective screening options. Based on this analysis Hemoccult II and flexible sigmoidoscopy are less attractive screening options because of the lower LYG with Hemoccult II and the lower LYG as well as the higher costs per life-year gained than other options with flexible sigmoidoscopy. CTC also is a less attractive strategy, with higher costs than other strategies that provide comparable or higher LYG at lower costs.

This CEA is also used to visualize and quantify the increase in costs per life-year gained when moving from one efficient strategy to the next highest strategy. The slope of the efficient frontier changes markedly from Hemoccult II to the Hemoccult SENSA strategy. Then there is a relatively flat line with only a slight increase in life-years saved relative to increasing costs for the remaining strategies. The inverse of the slope is used as the measure of the relative performance of the efficient strategies and is the incremental CER (ICER), defined as the additional cost of a specific strategy, divided by its additional clinical benefit, compared with the next least expensive strategy. For example, the incremental cost per life-year gained for the Hemoccult SENSA strategy relative to that of Hemoccult II is $16,605 per 1000 screened (see **Table 6**). The incremental cost per LYG is even higher going from the Hemoccult SENSA alone to the flexible sigmoidoscopy plus Hemoccult SENSA strategy ($73,336) and markedly higher in going from there to the flexible sigmoidoscopy plus FIT ($272,160). Those strategies on the flat of the efficient frontier curve represent diminishing returns of effectiveness per expenditure.[60]

The 2 strategies (DoD and ACRIN) for CTC are far from the efficient frontier when using a cost of $488 per scan for CTC, which is close to the $498 cost for colonoscopy without polypectomy. However, this value was a place-holder cost for CTC when assessing the conditions under which CTC could be cost-effective with the CRC screening tests currently reimbursed by CMS.[11,12] We used threshold analysis to determine that the cost per scan for CTC would have to be $108 to $122 (for the

CTC ACRIN and DoD strategies, respectively) in the 65-year-old cohort to place the CTC strategy on the efficient frontier (ie, thus cost-effective) relative to the LYG with the CTC strategy for the base case analysis. In a previous analysis using slightly different CTC test characteristics, Lansdorp-Vogelaar and colleagues[63] determined that CTC would need to be at a cost approximately 40% lower per scan than colonoscopy procedure with referral of CTC lesions 6 mm or larger and repeat CTC every 5 years to be cost-effective.

LIMITATIONS OF COST ESTIMATES

The costs of the screening tests, as well as the costs of complications associated with screening (primarily colonoscopy), were based on 2007 Medicare payment rates. To the extent that these rates change differentially in the future (eg, a decrease in the payment rate for colonoscopy) our results will change.

Costs for CRC treatment in this analysis were for the period 1998 to 2003 when the use of the expensive biologic therapies cetuximab and bevacizumab was limited.[64] We have used the MISCAN microsimulation modeling to project that with the increase in chemotherapy costs for treating advanced CRC, most CRC screening strategies provide cost savings by screening. (Colonoscopy does not become cost saving; however, the net costs of this strategy approach cost savings.[65])

SENSITIVITY ANALYSIS

An important component of CEA is the inclusion of sensitivity analysis on the base case assumptions of the model and costs. Lansdorp-Vogelaar and colleages[66] provide an example of a one-way and multivariate uncertainty analysis using a similar analysis as presented in this article. An important aspect of sensitivity analysis includes assessing the assumptions on adherence to the test strategy requirements (eg, annual FOBT or colonoscopy every 10 years).[40] The results given in this article are based on 100% adherence for all tests.

In this article we present the results from only one of the CISNET models as an example of CEA for these screening recommendations. A strength of the CISNET program is comparative modeling to provide a special type of sensitivity analysis of independently developed models addressing the same analysis. Similar results, and thus conclusions, were obtained by all 3 models, although the absolute values and rank orderings do differ.[11,12]

COST-EFFECTIVENESS SUMMARY

The CEA suggests that annual high sensitive FOBTs (guaiac and FIT), flexible sigmoidoscopy every 5 years with an annual sensitive FOBT, and colonoscopy are reasonable cost-effective screening strategies for CRC. Hemoccult II only and flexible sigmoidoscopy only are not included in this set of acceptable tests. Similarly, with current levels of test costs based on diagnostic procedures, CTC is not a cost-effective choice.

DO WE ACHIEVE THESE BENCHMARKS IN COMMUNITY PRACTICE?

To compare the common effectiveness of the screening procedures we first compared these tests with all having 100% adherence to all aspects of screening. However, in practice only 50% of those aged 50 years and older are compliant with current screening recommendations.[67,68] Those with no medical insurance, no regular source of care, and less education are less likely to receive CRC screening.[69] Furthermore, even in those having a positive screening test, there is nonadherence with follow-up diagnostic colonoscopy[70] and with surveillance colonoscopy for those with adenomas or CRC.[71] Also there is a decline in adherence for repeat FOBT testing.[72] In the decision analysis for the USPSTF, reducing adherence for colonoscopy screening from 100% to 80% reduced life-years saved by 20%, and reduction to 50% reduced colonoscopy life-years saved by 40%.[40] Nonadherence for initial screening, follow-up of positive tests or surveillance, and regular repeat screening affects screening interventions. To increase screening adherence we need interventions to increase both patient willingness to be screened as well as organizational structures within the medical system to facilitate identifying individuals in need of initial screening and to provide effective reminders for screening tests and follow-up. Physician recommendation is one of the most powerful incentives for individuals to be screened.[68]

The analysis presented here assumes that the colonoscopy for primary screening or for follow-up for a positive screening test is of high quality. This analysis includes a thorough examination of the colon based on good bowel preparation and reaching the cecum in 98% of cases. Effectiveness of the colonoscopy to prevent CRC can be compromised if colonoscopies do not achieve the standards as given by Standardized Colonoscopy Reporting and Data Systems (CO-RAD),[73,74] which include a benchmark of detection adenomas in 25% of men and 15% of women on screening colonoscopy. Kaminski and colleagues[75] have shown that endoscopists with higher adenoma detection rates had lower rates of interval cancers. The ACG has established quality indicators for colonoscopy, with a major focus on the quality of mucosal inspection and on obtaining safe and effective bowel preparation. Guidelines are given for an average of 6 minutes' withdrawal time from time of reaching the cecum. Attention to preventing complications is stressed with recommendations for hydration before, during, and after the procedure. Furthermore, continuing quality-evaluation programs are recommended for multiple specialty practices. A large gastrointestinal (GI) group in Minnesota has shown that the quality measures for CO-RADs can be monitored in the general GI practice using electronic records.[76]

New evidence from a randomized controlled trial of flexible sigmoidoscopy[77] shows that flexible sigmoidoscopy reduces the incidence for rectal and left-sided colon cancer but not for right-sided colon cancer. A case-control study from Canada[78] suggests that colonoscopy did not reduce right-sided colon cancer mortality. Further research is needed to determine the efficacy of colonoscopy for reducing right-sided disease and whether the biology or the possibilities of polypectomy intervention differ for the right and left colon.

CURRENT SCREENING GUIDELINES: DIFFERENCES AND COST IMPLICATIONS

This CEA supports a common theme of the 3 guideline groups that there are multiple acceptable CRC screening strategies. This analysis also identifies which screening tests are cost-effective given a range of willingness to pay per LYG. Furthermore, it is important that the patient has a choice in the decision of which test to use. The set of cost-effective strategies are annual sensitive FOBTs (either guaiac or FIT), flexible sigmoidoscopy every 5 years with a frequent sensitive FOBT, and colonoscopy (which is near the efficiency frontier). The CEA suggests that Hemoccult II, even though cost-effective, has a low LYG compared with the other screening strategies and would not be recommended given the willingness to pay in the United States. Also flexible sigmoidoscopy only every 5 years had lower LYG than other strategies with similar costs (and was dominated) and also would not be included as a recommended strategy. The ACS-MSTF-ACR and the ACG did not consider the combination of flexible sigmoidoscopy and sensitive FOBT, which was cost-effective and included in the menu of acceptable options by the USPSTF. Colonoscopy was only slightly more costly for its level of LYG than the flexible sigmoidoscopy plus FOBT strategies, which were on the efficient frontier. However, colonoscopy is one of the more expensive tests per LYG in the recommended cost-efficient screening strategies. In contrast, CTC would not be among the cost-effective strategies unless the cost per testing time was considerably less than that of colonoscopy and with referral of 6-mm polyps to colonoscopy with a 5-year repeat CTC.

The CEA was based on 100% adherence for all aspects of screening. In reality adherence is less overall and varies by screening test. Screening colonoscopy has increased rapidly in the past 5 years, whereas flexible sigmoidoscopy and FOBT have markedly decreased.[68] Availability of high-quality flexible sigmoidoscopies could be an issue if its use continues to diminish. The CEA suggested flexible sigmoidoscopy plus a sensitive FOBT would be cost-effective; however, this strategy requires the most test completion (considering flexible sigmoidoscopy every 5 years and an FOBT annually or biennially). Consequently, if adherence is low for either test, the overall effect of this strategy is altered.

The ACS-MSTF-ACR suggest favoring the cancer prevention CRC screening methods over those that primarily detected CRCs early. However, the CEAs suggest that the sensitive FOBTs had life-years saved almost comparable with those with colonoscopy given high adherence. If there is differential adherence with lower levels of adherence, including regular repeat screening for FOBTs, then the sensitive FOBTs would not attain similar LYG to those strategies that could prevent cancer. The role of adherence is key to understanding which CRC tests provide higher LYG at reasonable resource use and cost.

These results indicate that adherence to a strategy of screening is a critical component of saving life-years. The currently available screening tests provide substantial prevention for LYG and can be delivered within reasonable economic levels. Newer CRC screening tests need to be able to provide similar or higher levels of prevention, comparable levels of costs for screening, and high adherence.

REFERENCES

1. Winawer SJ, Fletcher RH, Miller L, et al. Colorectal cancer screening: clinical guidelines and rationale. Gastroenterology 1997;112(2):594–642.
2. Mandel J, Bond J, Church T, et al. Reducing mortality from colorectal cancer by screening for fecal occult blood. Minnesota Colon Cancer Control Study. N Engl J Med 1993;328(19):1365–71.
3. Hardcastle JD, Chamberlain JO, Robinson MH, et al. Randomised controlled trial of faecal-occult-blood screening for colorectal cancer. Lancet 1996;348(9040): 1472–7.
4. Kronborg O, Fenger C, Olsen J, et al. Randomised study of screening for colorectal cancer with faecal-occult-blood test. Lancet 1996;348(9040):1467–71.
5. Selby JV, Friedman GD, Quesenberry CP Jr, et al. A case-control study of screening sigmoidoscopy and mortality from colorectal cancer. N Engl J Med 1992;326(10):653–7.
6. Newcomb PA, Norfleet RG, Storer BE, et al. Screening sigmoidoscopy and colorectal cancer mortality. J Natl Cancer Inst 1992;84(20):1572–5.
7. Winawer SJ, Zauber AG, Ho MN, et al. Prevention of colorectal cancer by colonoscopic polypectomy. The National Polyp Study Workgroup. N Engl J Med 1993; 329(27):1977–81.

8. U.S. Preventive Services Task Force. Screening for colorectal cancer: U.S. Preventive Services Task Force recommendation statement. Ann Intern Med 2008;149(9):627–37.

9. Levin B, Lieberman DA, McFarland B, et al. Screening and surveillance for the early detection of colorectal cancer and adenomatous polyps, 2008: a joint guideline from the American Cancer Society, the US Multi-Society Task Force on Colorectal Cancer, and the American College of Radiology. Gastroenterology 2008;134(5):1570–95.

10. Rex DK, Johnson DA, Anderson JC, et al. American College of Gastroenterology guidelines for colorectal cancer screening 2009 [corrected]. Am J Gastroenterol 2009;104(3):739–50.

11. Zauber AG, Knudsen AB, Rutter CM, et al. Cost-effectiveness of CT colonography to screen for colorectal cancer. 2009. Available at: http://www1.cms.hhs. gov/mcd/viewtechassess.asp?from2=viewtechassess.asp&where=index&tid=58&. Accessed August 4, 2010.

12. Knudsen AB, Lansdorp-Vogelaar I, Rutter CM, et al. Cost-effectiveness of CT colonography screening for colorectal cancer in the medicare population. J Natl Cancer Inst 2010;102(16):1238–52.

13. Iglehart JK. Prioritizing comparative-effectiveness research–IOM recommendations. N Engl J Med 2009;361(4):325–8.

14. Van Gossum A, Munoz-Navas M, Fernandez-Urien I, et al. Capsule endoscopy versus colonoscopy for the detection of polyps and cancer. N Engl J Med 2009;361(3):264–70.

15. Bretthauer M. The capsule and colorectal-cancer screening–the crux of the matter. N Engl J Med 2009;361(3):300–1.

16. Pignone M, Saha S, Hoerger T, et al. Cost-effectiveness analyses of colorectal cancer screening: a systematic review for the U.S. Preventive Services Task Force. Ann Intern Med 2002;137(2):96–104.

17. Loeve F, Boer R, van Oortmarssen GJ, et al. The MISCAN-COLON simulation model for the evaluation of colorectal cancer screening. Comput Biomed Res 1999;32:13–33.

18. Frazier AL, Colditz GA, Fuchs CS, et al. Cost-effectiveness of screening for colorectal cancer in the general population. JAMA 2000;284(15):1954–61.

19. Ness RM, Holmes AM, Klein R, et al. Cost-utility of one-time colonoscopic screening for colorectal cancer at various ages. Am J Gastroenterol 2000; 95(7):1800–11.

20. Vijan S, Hwang EW, Hofer TP, et al. Which colon cancer screening test? A comparison of costs, effectiveness, and compliance. Am J Med 2001;111(8): 593–601.

21. Khandker RK, Dulski JD, Kilpatrick JB, et al. A decision model and cost-effectiveness analysis of colorectal cancer screening and surveillance guidelines for average-risk adults. Int J Technol Assess Health Care 2000;16(3): 799–810.

22. Pignone M, Rich M, Teutsch SM, et al. Screening for colorectal cancer in adults at average risk: a summary of the evidence for the U.S. Preventive Services Task Force. Ann Intern Med 2002;137(2):132–41.

23. Pignone M, Russell LB, Wagner JL. Economic models of colorectal cancer screening in average-risk. Washington, DC: National Academies Press; 2005.

24. Surveillance, Epidemiology, and End Results (SEER) Program (www.seer.cancer. gov) SEER*stat database: mortality- All COD, public-use with state, total U.S. (1969–2003), National Cancer Institute, DCCPS, Surveillance Research Program,

Cancer Statistics Branch, released April 2006. Underlying mortality data provided by NCHS (www.cdc.gov/nchs).

25. Clark JC, Collan Y, Eide TJ, et al. Prevalence of polyps in an autopsy series from areas with varying incidence of large-bowel cancer. Int J Cancer 1985;36(2): 179–86.

26. Blatt LJ. Polyps of the colon and rectum: incidence and distribution. Dis Colon Rectum 1961;4:277–82.

27. Arminski TC, McLean DW. Incidence and distribution of adenomatous polyps of the colon and rectum based on 1.000 autopsy examinations. Dis Colon Rectum 1964;7:249–61.

28. Vatn MH, Stalsberg H. The prevalence of polyps of the large intestine in Oslo: an autopsy study. Cancer 1982;49(4):819–25.

29. Jass JR, Young PJ, Robinson EM. Predictors of presence, multiplicity, size and dysplasia of colorectal adenomas. A necropsy study in New Zealand. Gut 1992;33:1508–14.

30. Johannsen LG, Momsen O, Jacobsen NO. Polyps of the large intestine in Aarhus, Denmark. An autopsy study. Scand J Gastroenterol 1989;24(7):799–806.

31. Bombi JA. Polyps of the colon in Barcelona, Spain. Cancer 1988;61(7):1472–6.

32. Williams AR, Balasooriya BA, Day DW. Polyps and cancer of the large bowel: a necropsy study in Liverpool. Gut 1982;23(10):835–42.

33. Rickert RR, Auerbach O, Garfinkel L, et al. Adenomatous lesions of the large bowel. Cancer 1979;43:1847–57.

34. Chapman I. Adenomatous polypi of large intestine: incidence and distribution. Ann Surg 1963;157:223–6.

35. Mandel JS, Church TR, Bond JH, et al. The effect of fecal occult-blood screening on the incidence of colorectal cancer. N Engl J Med 2000;343(22):1603–7.

36. Mandel JS, Church TR, Ederer F, et al. Colorectal cancer mortality: effectiveness of biennial screening for fecal occult blood. J Natl Cancer Inst 1999;91(5):434–7.

37. U.S. Preventive Services Task Force. Screening for colorectal cancer: recommendation and rationale. Ann Intern Med 2002;137(2):129–31.

38. Winawer SJ, Zauber AG, Fletcher RH, et al. Guidelines for colonoscopy surveillance after polypectomy: a consensus update by the US Multi-Society Task Force on Colorectal Cancer and the American Cancer Society. Published jointly in Gastroenterology 2006;130:1872–85 and CA Cancer J Clin 2006;56: 143–59.

39. van Ballegooijen M, Habbema JDF, Boer R, et al. Report to the Agency for Healthcare Research and Quality: a comparison of the cost-effectiveness of fecal occult blood tests with different test characteristics in the context of annual screening in the Medicare population. Available at: http://www.cms.gov/mcd/viewtechassess.asp?where=search&tid=20. Accessed August 4, 2010.

40. Zauber AG, Lansdorp-Vogelaar I, Knudsen AB, et al. Evaluating test strategies for colorectal cancer screening: a decision analysis for the U.S. Preventive Services Task Force. Ann Intern Med 2008;149(9):659–69.

41. Whitlock EP, Lin JS, Liles E, et al. Screening for colorectal cancer: a targeted, updated systematic review for the U.S. Preventive Services Task Force. Ann Intern Med 2008;149(9):638–58.

42. Hol L, van Leerdam ME, van Ballegooijen M, et al. Screening for colorectal cancer: randomised trial comparing guaiac-based and immunochemical faecal occult blood testing and flexible sigmoidoscopy. Gut 2010;59(1):62–8.

43. Mulhall BP, Veerappan GR, Jackson JL. Meta-analysis: computed tomographic colonography. Ann Intern Med 2005;142(8):635–50.

44. Doria-Rose VP, Levin TR, Selby JV, et al. The incidence of colorectal cancer following a negative screening sigmoidoscopy: implications for screening interval. Gastroenterology 2004;127(3):714–22.

45. Adam I, Ali Z, Shorthouse A. How accurate is the endoscopist's assessment of visualization of the left colon seen at flexible sigmoidoscopy? Colorectal Dis 2001;2(1):41–4.

46. Pickhardt PJ, Choi JR, Hwang I, et al. Computed tomographic virtual colonoscopy to screen for colorectal neoplasia in asymptomatic adults. N Engl J Med 2003;349(23):2191–200.

47. Johnson CD, Chen MH, Toledano AY, et al. Accuracy of CT colonography for detection of large adenomas and cancers. N Engl J Med 2008;359(12):1207–17.

48. Zauber AG, Lansdorp-Vogelaar I, Wilschut J, et al. Cost-effectiveness of DNA stool testing to screen for colorectal cancer: report to AHRQ and CMS from the Cancer Intervention and Surveillance Modeling Network (CISNET) for MISCAN and SimCRC Models. Available at: https://www.cms.hhs.gov/mcd/viewtechassess.asp?from2=viewtechassess.asp&id=212&. Accessed August 4, 2010.

49. Levin TR, Zhao W, Conell C, et al. Complications of colonoscopy in an integrated health care delivery system. Ann Intern Med 2006;145(12):880–6.

50. Lieberman DA, Weiss DG, Bond JH, et al. Use of colonoscopy to screen asymptomatic adults for colorectal cancer. Veterans Affairs Cooperative Study Group 380. N Engl J Med 2000;343(3):162–8.

51. Pox C, Schmiegel W, Classen M. Current status of screening colonoscopy in Europe and in the United States. Endoscopy 2007;39(2):168–73.

52. Klabunde CN, Warren JL, Ransohoff DF, et al. Complications of colonoscopy in the Medicare population. Gastroenterology 2007;132(Suppl 2):A149 (995).

53. Warren JL, Klabunde CN, Mariotto AB, et al. Adverse events after outpatient colonoscopy in the Medicare population. Ann Intern Med 2009;150(12):849–57, W152.

54. Regula J, Rupinski M, Kraszewska E, et al. Colonoscopy in colorectal-cancer screening for detection of advanced neoplasia. N Engl J Med 2006;355(18):1863–72.

55. Levin TR, Conell C, Shapiro JA, et al. Complications of screening flexible sigmoidoscopy. Gastroenterology 2002;123(6):1786–92.

56. Ko CW, Riffle S, Michaels L, et al. Serious complications within 30 days of screening and surveillance colonoscopy are uncommon. Clin Gastroenterol Hepatol 2010;8(2):166–73.

57. Rabeneck L, Paszat LF, Hilsden RJ, et al. Bleeding and perforation after outpatient colonoscopy and their risk factors in usual clinical practice. Gastroenterology 2008;135(6):1899–906, 1906, e1891.

58. Yabroff KR, Lamont EB, Mariotto A, et al. Cost of care for elderly cancer patients in the United States. J Natl Cancer Inst 2008;100(9):630–41.

59. Brown ML, Riley GF, Schussler N, et al. Estimating health care costs related to cancer treatment from SEER-Medicare data. Med Care 2002;40(8 Suppl):IV-104–17.

60. Mark DH. Visualizing cost-effectiveness analysis. JAMA 2002;287(18):2428–9.

61. Petitti DB. In: Meta-analysis, decision analysis, and cost-effectiveness analysis: methods for quantitative synthesis in medicine, vol. 31. 2nd edition. New York: Oxford University Press; 2000.

62. Gold MR, Siegel JE, Russell LB, et al. Cost-effectiveness in health and medicine. New York: Oxford University Press; 1996.

63. Lansdorp-Vogelaar I, van Ballegooijen M, Zauber AG, et al. At what costs will screening with CT colonography be competitive? A cost-effectiveness approach. Int J Cancer 2009;124(5):1161–8.

64. Schrag D. The price tag on progress–chemotherapy for colorectal cancer. N Engl J Med 2004;351(4):317–9.

65. Lansdorp-Vogelaar I, van Ballegooijen M, Zauber AG, et al. Effect of rising chemotherapy costs on the cost savings of colorectal cancer screening. J Natl Cancer Inst 2009;101(20):1412–22.

66. Lansdorp-Vogelaar I, van Ballegooijen M, Zauber AG, et al. Individualizing colonoscopy screening by sex and race. Gastrointest Endosc 2009;70(1):96–108, 108, e101–124.

67. Shapiro JA, Seeff LC, Thompson TD, et al. Colorectal cancer test use from the 2005 National Health Interview Survey. Cancer Epidemiol Biomarkers Prev 2008;17(7):1623–30.

68. NIH State-of-the-Science Conference: enhancing use and quality of colorectal cancer screening. Bethesda, MA, February 2–4, 2010. Available at: http://www.consensus.nih.gov/2010/colorectalstatement.htm. Accessed August 4, 2010.

69. Coups EJ, Manne SL, Meropol NJ, et al. Multiple behavioral risk factors for colorectal cancer and colorectal cancer screening status. Cancer Epidemiol Biomarkers Prev 2007;16(3):510–6.

70. Miglioretti DL, Rutter CM, Bradford SC, et al. Improvement in the diagnostic evaluation of a positive fecal occult blood test in an integrated health care organization. Med Care 2008;46(9 Suppl 1):S91–6.

71. Schoen RE, Pinsky PF, Weissfeld JL, et al. Utilization of surveillance colonoscopy in community practice. Gastroenterology 2010;138(1):73–81.

72. Weller D, Coleman D, Robertson R, et al. The UK colorectal cancer screening pilot: results of the second round of screening in England. Br J Cancer 2007;97(12):1601–5.

73. Rex DK, Petrini JL, Baron TH, et al. Quality indicators for colonoscopy. Am J Gastroenterol 2006;101(4):873–85.

74. Lieberman D. A call to action–measuring the quality of colonoscopy. N Engl J Med 2006;355(24):2588–9.

75. Kaminski MF, Regula J, Kraszewska E, et al. Quality indicators for colonoscopy and the risk of interval cancer. N Engl J Med 2010;362(19):1795–803.

76. Shaukat A, Oancea C, Bond JH, et al. Variation in detection of adenomas and polyps by colonoscopy and change over time with a performance improvement program. Clin Gastroenterol Hepatol 2009;7(12):1335–40.

77. Atkin WS, Edwards R, Kralj-Hans I, et al. Once-only flexible sigmoidoscopy screening in prevention of colorectal cancer: a multicentre randomised controlled trial. Lancet 2010;375(9726):1624–33.

78. Baxter NN, Goldwasser MA, Paszat LF, et al. Association of colonoscopy and death from colorectal cancer. Ann Intern Med 2009;150(1):1–8.

79. Pickhardt PJ, Lee AD, Taylor AJ, et al. Primary 2D versus primary 3D polyp detection at screening CT colonography. AJR Am J Roentgenol 2007;189(6):1451–6.

Maximizing the Value of Colonoscopy in Community Practice

John I. Allen, MD, MBA, AGAF[a,b]

KEYWORDS

- Colonoscopy • Community endoscopy • Colonoscopy quality
- Colorectal cancer prevention
- Colorectal cancer screening costs • Screening
- Quality of colonoscopy • Value of colonoscopy

The value of a medical service is defined as the incremental increase in health per unit cost. The value equation is generally written as follows:

HEALTH VALUE = QUALITY/COST

Quality, in this context, reflects the Institute of Medicine's 6 Aims for health care, which focus on safety, timeliness, effectiveness, efficacy, and equitable patient-centered care. *Cost* can be defined at a patient (episode cost) or population level.

In 1998, colonoscopy became a covered benefit for Medicare patients when used for colorectal cancer (CRC) screening.[1] Medicare coverage spurred commercial health plans to implement a similar benefit and by now colonoscopy has become the community standard for CRC screening and is most frequently advocated in both scientific and lay press.[2,3]

A screening test, by definition, is recommended for a large segment of the population that shows no signs or symptoms of the condition in question. As such, the test must be effective, safe, resource efficient, and widely available. Of all tests included in the US Preventative Services Task Force (USPSTF) *Guide to Adult Clinical Preventive Services*, colonoscopy is the most invasive, expensive, and dangerous. When gastroenterologists led the effort to have screening colonoscopy covered, collectively we made an implicit promise to maximize its health value and build infrastructure needed to provide it.

As of 2010, between 10 and 12 million patients undergo colonoscopy annually in the United States and the 10,000 board-certified, community-based gastroenterologists currently practicing perform most of the examinations. Therefore, it is essential that

No grant support and no disclosures.
a Minnesota Gastroenterology PA, PO Box 14909, Minneapolis, MN 55414, USA
b University of Minnesota School of Medicine, 420 Delaware Street, SE, Minneapolis, MN 55455, USA
E-mail address: jallen@mngastro.com

we try and determine if the value of these examinations has been pushed to their maximal extent. This article discusses the value of community-based colonoscopy, a term that includes both quality and cost.

HISTORICAL CONSIDERATIONS OF SCREENING COLONOSCOPY

Scientific evidence supporting the effectiveness of colonoscopy to reduce CRC came from the National Polyp Study (NPS) published in 1993.[4] The authors concluded that a high-quality colonoscopy that cleared the colon of all neoplastic lesions would reduce risk of CRC by 76% to 90%, with subsequent analysis suggesting an effect sustained for at least 10 years. Based on these findings and several smaller, feasibility studies, the Health Care Financing Administration (HCFA, subsequently known as the Center for Medicare and Medicaid [CMS]) elected to cover colonoscopy for average-risk beneficiaries. Subsequently, USPSTF gave CRC screening (including colonoscopy) a Grade A recommendation.

Once scientific evidence exists to support a population-based screening test, a cost-benefit ratio is calculated and compared with other interventions that are covered benefits. Screening tests were often compared with the cost (per year of life saved) of renal dialysis, which the government had agreed to cover under Public Law 92-603 in 1972. In 1998, the cost per year of life saved by colonoscopy screening was estimated to be about $15,000, less than that of dialysis and breast cancer screening, for example. In 2000, Sonnenberg and colleagues[5] concluded, "Colonoscopy represents a cost-effective means of screening for colorectal cancer because it reduces mortality at relatively low incremental costs." Recently, Zauber and colleagues[6] published a decision analysis of multiple CRC screening strategies for the USPSTF and an updated cost-effectiveness analysis for the Agency for Health care Research and Quality.[7]

It is important to review the underlying assumptions of these publications because they reflect the generally accepted cost benefit for colonoscopy. Sonnenberg's cost-effectiveness analysis assumed a 75% reduction in CRC risk with colonoscopy at a per-procedure cost of $681 for a screening examination (45,378) and $1000 for a colonoscopy that included polypectomy (45,385). Sensitivity analysis revealed that a reduction in efficacy of colonoscopy to 60% doubled the overall cost. Zauber's analyses concluded that colonoscopy was the most effective screening test based on a 95% sensitivity of colonoscopy for advanced polyps and cancer with a per-procedure cost of $800 for 45,378 and $1000 for 45,385.

QUALITY ISSUES FOR COLONOSCOPY IN 2010

Since these original estimates, several changes have occurred that affect the value of colonoscopy. There is clear evidence that the quality of colonoscopy examinations in the general community is variable, many practices (both primary care and specialists) do not follow evidence-based screening and surveillance guidelines (leading to both overuse and underuse), colonoscopy's CRC risk reduction appears to be less than originally thought, and the total cost of CRC screening has increased substantially. Each of these points are discussed further.

Recent publications have brought into question the effectiveness of community-based colonoscopy as a CRC prevention modality likely because training and credentialing of community endoscopists varies and quality is generally not monitored. One large, retrospective outcome study suggested that colonoscopy provides a risk reduction of approximately 65% and most (if not all) of the effect applies to left-sided cancers.[8] Although this study has methodological weaknesses, findings suggest that

NPS conclusions were either overly optimistic or that community-based physicians do not generate results that match NPS investigators. Factors known to compromise efficacy include missed prevalent cancers (incomplete examinations or true visual misses), missed proximal precancerous polyps (which tend to grow in a sessile or flat configuration), underestimation of the cancer potential of proximal serrated lesions (usually by the pathologist), microsatellite instable polyps that are difficult to resect fully and tend to grow rapidly, small flat adenomas, rapid examination times, and a variety of other factors.[9,10]

Miss rates for CRC among endoscopists vary 10-fold from 0.5% to 5.0%[11,12] and from 6% to 18% for adenomas greater than 5 mm.[13] Barclay and colleagues[14] studied the relation between an endoscopist's withdrawal time (time from cecum to examination end) and their adenoma find rate (AFR), which is defined as the percentage of average risk patients in whom at least 1 adenoma was discovered during a screening examination. They demonstrated significant differences in AFR between endoscopists with a withdrawal time less than 6 minutes compared with those whose withdrawal times exceeded 6 minutes. They then demonstrated an increase in AFR among experienced colonoscopists by using an audible timer to slow examiners.[15]

Others have emphasized the relationship between adenoma detection at colonoscopy and factors, such as preparation quality, level of sedation, and total procedure time.[16,17] Withdrawal time measurement has become a common surrogate measure for colonoscopy quality, but 2 subsequent studies demonstrated that factors other than increasing withdrawal time will be needed to improve adenoma detection among those endoscopists who have low baseline detection rates.[18,19]

Variation in colonoscopy quality and outcomes exists and will likely continue until process and outcome measures for all colonoscopy examinations are either mandated (see later discussion) or become a routine part of practice for both gastroenterologists and nongastroenterologists who perform screening colonoscopy. The current system of fee-for-service reimbursement, which is disconnected from health outcomes, and credentialing of endoscopists at the facility level (a situation with inherent economic conflicts of interest) both suggest that factors other than quality and patient-centered health outcomes will continue to be powerful influences in community settings.

COST ISSUES IN COLONOSCOPY IN 2010

In the last decade, the cost for CRC prevention has exploded in the United States, a factor that by itself has the potential to diminish the value of colonoscopy to society. Careful analysis of factors driving this cost increase help us understand if this trend can be slowed.

Before 1998, the percentage of Medicare recipients who underwent any type of CRC screening was estimated to be approximately 25% and most were screened using fecal occult blood tests.[1] Screening rates are now approximately 50% and most people undergo colonoscopy. This trend has paralleled a 2% annual decrease in CRC incidence over 2 decades, a change thought to be attributable in large part to screening and polyp removal. Annually, there are 10 to 12 million colonoscopy examinations in the United States with approximately 75% performed for CRC screening or surveillance. It is estimated that if screening rates were to increase to 70% of eligible Americans, an additional 10 million colonoscopy examinations would be needed. Ten million examinations at an average cost of $800 would translate to a national cost of $8 billion annually. As demonstrated in the following discussion, this is certainly an underestimate.

In 1980, Medicare reimbursed colonoscopy at a rate of approximately $500 for the professional fee (with regional variation) and $2000 for the facility fee (colonoscopy was universally performed in a hospital setting). In 1983, the first Medicare Certified Ambulatory Endoscopy Center (AEC) opened in Tennessee, followed 2 months later by one in Minnesota. Shortly thereafter, for-profit companies emerged offering to partner with physicians in building AECs.[20] The subsequent increase in AECs is well documented and there are now more than 5100 Medicare-certified centers in the United States. These centers, for the most part, were built by community-based gastroenterologists and provide the major infrastructure needed to deliver on our CRC prevention commitment.

Profitability from managing an AEC is still acceptable, although stringent regulations and increasing fixed costs are leading many physicians to sell AECs to hospitals in a joint-venture arrangement. Despite financial and managerial obstacles over the last decade, the proliferation of accessible, cost-effective AECs led to the vast expansion of CRC screening capability in the United States and hastened the widespread use of colonoscopy as the primary CRC screening test.

In addition to overall increases in the volume of colonoscopy, per-procedure costs have escalated dramatically despite moving most examinations from hospitals to AECs. Colonoscopy, as practiced today, can be delivered in a hospital outpatient department (HOPD), an AEC, or an office. Both HOPD and AECs receive a facility fee (CMS AEC facility fees are now tied to HOPD at approximately 65%). Office endoscopy does not generate a separate facility fee but the professional fee paid by CMS is augmented to cover increased office expense of the service (site of service differential). In addition, sedation might be administered by the endoscopy team (no additional payment) or an anesthesia professional (separate charge). Entire costs for a screening colonoscopy might include some or all of the following: (1) preprocedure evaluation (not covered by CMS for screening examinations), (2) endoscopist professional fee, (3) facility fee (hospital or AEC), (4) pathology facility charge (if biopsies are sent), (5) pathology professional charge, (6) anesthesia professional fee, (8) costs of complications, (9) cost of ancillary examinations (imaging for incomplete procedures), and (10) indirect costs (lost work for both patients and their ride). Widespread practice changes that add to any portion of the per-unit cost will lead to a substantial escalation of the nation's total cost of CRC prevention and diminish overall value unless there is a demonstrable increase in quality or health outcomes.

Patients undergoing colonoscopy in HOPD are subjected to an unbundled facility charge where equipment costs are passed along as line items. In AECs, all equipment is bundled into the facility fee, thus making future predictions of costs more accurate. HOPD charges are frequently 2 to 10 times more than the charges from an AEC.

The actual per-procedure cost of colonoscopy is not generally known or publicized. On the Minnesota Gastroenterology Web site, the cost of a screening colonoscopy is listed as $1568 (professional and facility fee only). Atlanta Gastroenterology (Atlanta, Georgia) charges a bundled fee of $1500 for cash-pay (or high deductible) patients, which includes the endoscopist's professional fee, facility, pathology, and anesthesia.[21] It should be noted that the listed fee at the author's organization (and likely that of the Atlanta group) represents a financial target that is based on regional reimbursement and the estimated impact of the fee on the small proportion of cash-based patients. In reality, insurance-based reimbursement unbundles the charges and depends on negotiated rates for each component of service. Thus, facility fees can range from $346 (Medicare) to more than $5000. The upper end reflects commercial payers that must negotiate HOPD rates as part of a total health delivery contract, often with hospitals that enjoy enhanced bargaining power because of geographic imperatives or a reputation as a must-have facility. Similarly, anesthesia professionals might cost less than $200 per case (Medicare) or more than $1000 for anesthesiologists that do not participate in a particular patient's health plan (non-par). Less dramatic fluctuations in price occur for endoscopy professional fees and pathology.

In 2009, Minnesota Gastroenterology performed 36,031 colonoscopy procedures in their AECs (**Table 1**), for a total annual cost to Minnesota payers of approximately $60,000,000 (including all of the direct medical costs listed previously). The increase in pathology rates (see **Table 1**) alone, compared with 2006, increased cost by $1.8 million. If they were to close all AECs and perform colonoscopy within the regional HOPDs, where average facility fees would add approximately $850 per procedure, the annual increased cost for this change alone would be $30,626,350. If anesthesia professionals administered sedation in their AECs, it would add approximately $350 (conservatively) to each procedure for an annual increase of $12,610,850 (colonoscopy alone, not including upper endoscopy). If they made both changes, and used HOPD anesthesia, the increase in cost for the same physicians performing colonoscopy on the same patients would be approximately $57,000,000 annually, which is about double the current cost (see previous discussion). Remember, 10 to 12 million colonoscopy examinations are performed annually and we are advocating for 10 million more (increased screening rates).

Nationally, there are increasing trends to close AECs and move patients to HOPDs because of increased costs of running AECs. CMS has been criticized for lax survey and credentialing standards based on a widely publicized infection control disaster in Las Vegas Nevada in 2008 within a certified AEC. Subsequent spot surveys of other Medicare-certified AECs revealed that safety concerns similar to those found in Las Vegas were widespread (personal communication with the Survey and Certification Unit of CMS). The response of CMS has been to increase regulations and survey intensity. This recent action, combined with imminent threat of sanctions by Recovery Audit Contractors, has increased the cost and financial risk of managing centers to a level sufficient to drive some physician-owners to sell their AEC to regional hospitals. This trend will increase costs because procedure facility fees then rise to HOPD rates. Concurrently, the percentage of endoscopy procedures performed with sedation provided by an anesthesia professional now approaches 50% nationally. In the last 5 years, all increases in per-procedure costs for colonoscopy have been directed to

Table 1 Colonoscopy statistics from Minnesota Gastroenterology-owned AEC's from 2004 through 2009						
	2004	2005	2006	2007	2008	2009
Number of examinations	27,253	33,995	35,099	37,817	36,972	36,031
Complete (%)	97	98	98	97	97	97
Path sent (%)	39	43	35	41	52	54
AFR: male (%)	28	32	26	30	32	40
AFR: female (%)	18	21	17	19	22	28
>6 minute withdrawal (%)	NM	NM	NM	76	95	99

Number of exams performed (all by Board Certified Gastroenterologists). Path sent refers to the % of colonoscopy exams where one or more biopsy specimens were sent. AFR for males or females 50 years of age and older during a screening or surveillance examination. Withdrawal time is measured from the point the endoscope passes the ileal cecal valve until exit from the anus.
Abbreviations: AFR, adenoma find rate; NM, not measured.

hospitals and anesthesiologists. Payment to gastroenterologists has fallen substantially because of reduced professional and facility fees (mostly by Medicare).

There is no evidence from controlled trials that performing a colonoscopy in an HOPD versus AEC or adding an anesthesia professional impacts outcomes for healthy patients undergoing CRC screening. Until valid outcomes research is performed to answer these questions (see later discussion regarding Digestive Health Outcomes Registry), we cannot conclude that we are adding value compared with practices using an AEC and conscious sedation.

Besides an increase in per-procedure cost, increases in the annual volume of colonoscopy have impacted total health costs. In 2008, the author's organization analyzed the actual total direct costs of 27,253 colonoscopy examinations performed in our AECs during 2004. These were examinations performed without preprocedure consultation, under conscious sedation, where 39% of examinations included a biopsy, 97% were complete (few ancillary imaging examinations), and there were 30 serious complications (22 emergency department visits alone and 8 requiring hospitalization). Their cancer miss rate (defined as within 3 years of a colonoscopy) for 2004 was 6 known cases (as reported publically in their 2008 outcomes booklet). The cancer misses were not included in the financial analysis. The direct cost (dollars paid, not charges) for all preprocedure, intraprocedure, and postprocedure services was just less than $30,000,000. As calculated previously, that number is now $60,000,000, based on 36,031 examinations performed in 2009 with similar practice patterns.

More colonoscopy examinations should be hailed as a triumph because screening rates appear to have increased. Unfortunately, evidence for overuse and misuse of surveillance colonoscopy has tempered our celebration.[22,23] Both gastroenterologists and primary care physicians fail to follow CRC screening and surveillance guidelines for a variety of reasons as outlined in a recent editorial in *Gastroenterology*.[20]

Although it is difficult for us to admit, it appears that the value of colonoscopy is less than we thought in 1998, when Medicare began covering screening colonoscopy. This apparent reduction in the value of colonoscopy as a CRC prevention measure has occurred despite medical-society–generated guidelines, physician education, research advances, improved scope technology, more comfortable patients (no one denies propofol is a better sedative than opioids and midazolam), and public campaigns to increase screening rates.

ALTERNATIVE APPROACHES TO ENHANCING VALUE OF COLONOSCOPY

In 2010, a 50-year-old patient needing a screening colonoscopy can be referred to a physician who has an AFR of 7% and receive a bill for more than $5000 or to a physician in the same area whose AFR is 45% and receive a bill for $900. The following initiatives are designed to alter this situation:

- Practice level quality and price transparency
- State initiatives
- Bundled payments
- Digestive Health Outcomes Registry.

PRACTICE LEVEL QUALITY AND PRICE TRANSPARENCY

Practice level price transparency has been previously discussed and remains extremely rare nationwide. Quality measurement by practices is becoming more widespread, although public reporting of results is still unusual. In 2004, the physicians of Minnesota Gastroenterology began a performance-improvement initiative focused on colonoscopy developed in conjunction with their implementing an electronic medical record. The program has been described in detail elsewhere.[19,24] Since 2004, the following data were collected for each physician: (1) number of colonoscopy examinations performed annually, (2) completion rate (documented to the end of the colon), (3) AFR by gender, for both screening examinations alone and combined with surveillance examinations, (there was no difference in rates so these were combined in subsequent analyses), (4) percentage of examinations where pathology specimens were submitted, and (5) complication data (as described by Allen,[24] but not presented here).

From 2004 until 2007, 5 specific interventions designed to improve AFR were implemented, including presentation of data blinded to physician, physician-identified data, educational seminars about quality improvement, individual discussions with physicians having low AFR, and finally financial incentives to achieve a withdrawal time greater than 6 minutes for more than 95% of all examinations. In 2008 and 2009 more financial incentives were attached to withdrawal time, further individual discussions occurred with partners that continued to have low AFR, each of whom were asked to undergo an eye examination and watch learning videos. **Table 1** is a summary of practice-level data from 2004 to 2009 (inclusive).

More than 85% of patients referred to the author's practice for colonoscopy examinations were distributed randomly to partners (15% are referrals to specific physicians and gender preferences are respected). The numerical range of colonoscopy examinations per partner varied from 92 per year to 1348 (2009 data). Women partners (n = 8) tended to have more women patients than male partners (average: 65% compared with 48%). All examinations were performed using opioid and midazolam conscious sedation. The author's practice consistently has a sedation reversal rate (use of reversal agents) of approximately 0.3% and in 27 years of operation, there have been no in-center deaths. Complications are reported to a secure practice phone line and are reviewed within a legally codified peer-review process. Complication rates are well within reported ranges and are published in their annual outcomes booklet[24] (also available at www.mngastro.com).

Overall, AFR per physicians adjusted for age, sex, and adequate preparation quality varied from 10% to 39% from 2005 to 2007 (both genders combined).[19] It should be noted that the term *AFR* in the author's practice refers to all precancerous polyps, not just traditional adenomas (sessile serrated adenomas, for example). AFR plotted for individual physicians over time (2004–2007) showed no patterns or trends, despite the educational programs and feedback. Variation for an individual physician was random, suggesting that physicians tended to have a constant rate of AFR and the applied interventions were ineffective in changing rates during the 3-year study period.

AFR was only correlated strongly with the percent of examinations where pathology was submitted. In February 2007, the practice opened a pathology laboratory where biopsy specimens were processed internally; whereas, professional interpretation was performed by an independent group of pathologists and billed separately. As can be appreciated from **Table 1**, the rate that pathology was submitted from colonoscopy increased from 35% in 2006 to 54% in 2009. In addition, increased individual attention paid to physicians with a low AFR appeared to have paid off, because by 2009 all physicians were above the published threshold for AFR for both men (25%) and women (15%). Overall, practice AFR increased to 40% for men and 28% for women.

Their 6-year experience of closely monitoring colonoscopy quality measures was discouraging for the first 4 years because it appeared that experienced endoscopists could not alter their AFR despite education and best individual efforts. At year 5 and 6, however, there was a sustained increase in AFR for all physicians. It is not clear what factor was most powerful in driving AFR. Withdrawal times were increased in early 2008, but the dramatic increase in AFR did not occur until 2009. Whatever worked, it appears that measuring quality within a practice committed to improvement and supported by strong peer governance paid off in measureable improvements.

STATE INITIATIVES

Changes in colonoscopy quality nationally will require a more coordinated effort than is available within single practices. State-level initiatives are now being implemented to enhance quality and to drive price transparency. Minnesota is a unique state because companies that provide medical insurance have to be a nonprofit, Minnesota-based, state-certified company. This situation has provided opportunities for state-level collaboration, such as Minnesota Community Measurement (MCM), a nonprofit organization created 6 years ago to measure practice-level clinical outcomes. Seven nonprofit health benefit companies licensed in Minnesota support MCM financially and the state medical society is a founding member. The Minnesota Department of Health has representation on the MCM Board. MCM has published practice-level clinical outcomes since 2005 for 300 primary care clinics (90% of primary care in Minnesota; see www.mnhealthscores.org).

In 2009, MCM began developing measures for specialty care with colonoscopy targeted as the first initiative. A task force of primary care providers, administrators, and specialists met over a 6-month period to develop valid measures. Data collection begins in July 2010 on a voluntary basis, but the Minnesota Department of Health has indicated that it may require participation in 2011 as a prerequisite for payment. Several large physician-hospital systems have indicated that they intend to refer patients for colonoscopy examinations only to providers that participate in quality measurement.

Measures will be collected at a physician level, but public reporting will begin at a clinic or practice level, which may change in the future. The exact reporting methodology is still under debate and will be determined by an expert panel as data begins to accumulate. For example, exact AFR may not be listed, but the public report might indicate an AFR above or below acceptable levels. Specific measures will be as follows:

1. Total number of colonoscopy examinations performed annually (validated by claims analysis)
2. Completion rate
3. Number of examinations in average risk, screen patients where a precancerous polyp is found (based on pathology results)
4. Ten-year interval recommended for low-risk patients (no precancerous polyps at colonoscopy)
5. Appropriate surveillance recommendation for higher-risk patients (based on guidelines).

MCM has previously developed a registry function, methodology for direct data submission (DDS), and a random audit process to validate submitted information. All but a few endoscopists work within a HOPD already able to provide DDS to MCM. Physicians that do not perform HOPD-based colonoscopy (Minnesota Gastroenterology, for example) will create a new electronic interface with MCM. It is anticipated that the majority of physicians who perform colonoscopy in Minnesota will be participating by 2011. The author knows of at least one other state that has a similar initiative (New Hampshire). It will be interesting to see if the improvements noted at the author's practice level will be duplicated when statewide reporting begins and results are made public.

BUNDLED PAYMENT METHODOLOGIES

Value-based reimbursement is beginning to emerge in multiple markets. Here, providers accept payments bundled around clinical episodes of care and assume some portion of either performance or insurance risk. Providers that improve quality or reduce costs are rewarded with enhanced fees. Two projects known to the author have defined episodes of colonoscopy screening care based on procedural and diagnosis codes. The High Value Health care Project funded by Robert Woods Johnson (described in the article by Brennan and colleagues elsewhere in this issue) seeks to build a fully transparent cost of care infrastructure so that real comparisons among providers of services can develop. Brennan and colleagues detail their method of developing episodes and discuss the implications for gastroenterology.

The Prometheus project follows a similar methodology to bundle colonoscopy services, but adds a risk-sharing payment mechanism.[25] This method of payment defines expected versus unexpected results for service episodes (called "Potentially Avoidable Complications" or PACs). Incentives are based on resources used for the underlying service plus reduction in PACs. Each reimbursement cycle (usually annual) requires meeting increasingly stringent targets for incentive payments.

A step beyond episode bundling occurs with development of accountable care organizations (ACO), which are health delivery systems that assume both financial and clinical risk for total cost of care for a population. One experiment with ACOs is a tricity pilot based on a model defined by Fisher and colleagues.[26] Pilots are being funded by health benefit companies and involve virtually integrated care systems working in conjunction with a payer who provides claims analysis. Current ACO iterations differ from capitated plans of the 1990s, because reimbursement remains as traditional fee for service but the total budget (usually 3 years) is predicated on 3 years past claims (plus actuarial and cost of living increases). Savings generated by system-wide coordination of care (reduction in rehospitalization rates, for example) and success in bending the cost curve result in savings shared equally by providers and purchasers.

DIGESTIVE HEALTH OUTCOMES REGISTRY

Digestive health outcomes registry is an initiative jointly developed by the American Gastroenterological Association Institute and MedAssurant Inc, a company specializing in health care data aggregation and analysis. The purpose of this registry is to give practices an ability to measure quality outcomes and manage care at a population level (see www.agaregistry.org). One initial topic will be CRC prevention, including colonoscopy. Measures, such as screening rates, colonoscopy quality, resource use, use of anesthesia professionals, site of service, and surveillance recommendations, will be reported monthly to participating practices and aggregated at a national level. Comparisons can be made against like practices, regional providers, academic medical centers, or the entire spectrum of practices. The newly created gastrointestinal registry will be prepopulated from an existing database, maintained by MedAssurant Inc, containing more than 2 billion patient encounters. From these data, we will be able to discern differences in outcomes from working with anesthesiologists or performing procedures in an HOPD versus AEC. By definition, an outcomes registry is an observational methodology that reflects practice in usual community care (as opposed to a controlled research study). Other specialty registries, such as cardiology, bariatric surgery, oncology, rheumatology, and orthopedics, have driven improvements in care at a national level. The development of national outcome registries might speed quality improvement by facilitating aggregate-level incentives, such as those described by Mandel.[27]

SUMMARY

What are the implications of these initiatives for national colonoscopy improvement efforts? Bluntly stated, the commitment of the United States to CRC prevention is huge and providers who provide screening examinations should be held accountable for results and work to maximize the value of colonoscopy to the patients we see and to society as a whole. A commitment to enhancing value means a commitment to improving quality (known to be variable) and reducing total cost of care. Because we (gastroenterologists) led the effort to mandate population-based CRC screening with colonoscopy, we have an ethical commitment to be vigilant about our results and accountable for outcomes.

Gastroenterologists who understand future reimbursement and health care trends are already preparing their practice infrastructure to meet new challenges of transparency and bundled payments. Market-based pressures derived from quality and cost transparency will be sufficient to drive change. Robust measurement and public reporting of results are both firmly embedded in some regions of the country and will spread nationally within the next few years. The path is clear for those who study these issues; monitor process measures for internal improvement, push resource efficiency, connect to national registries to demonstrate quality externally, and constantly try to provide a service with the highest health value.

REFERENCES

1. Heinrickf J. Beneficiary use of clinical preventive services. United States General Accounting Office Report; 2002. Available at: http://www.gao.gov/products/GAO-02-777T. Accessed February 23, 2010.
2. Lieberman DA. Screening for colorectal cancer. N Engl J Med 2009;361:1179–87.
3. Katz ML, Sheridan S, Pignone M, et al. Prostate and colon cancer screening messages in popular magazines. J Gen Intern Med 2004;19:843–8.
4. Winawer SJ, Zauber AG, Ho MN, et al. Prevention of colorectal cancer by colonoscopic polypectomy. N Engl J Med 1993;329:1977–81.
5. Sonnenberg A, Fabiola D, Inadomi JM. Cost-effectiveness of colonoscopy in screening for colorectal cancer. Ann Intern Med 2000;133:573–84.
6. Zauber AG, Lansdorp-Vogelaar I, Knudsen AB, et al. Evaluating test strategies for colorectal cancer screening: a decision analysis for the US Preventative Services Task Force. Ann Intern Med 2008;149:659–69.
7. Zauber AG, Lansdorp-Vogelaar I, Wilschut J, et-al. Cost-effectiveness of DNA stool testing to screen for colorectal cancer: report to AHRQ and CMS from the Cancer Intervention and Surveillance Modeling Network (CISNET) for MISCAN and SimCRC Models. Available at: https://www.cms.hhs.gov/mcd/viewtechassess.asp?from2=viewtechassess.asp&id=212&.asp&id=212&. Accessed February 24, 2010.
8. Baxter NN, Goldwasser MA, Paszat LF, et al. Association of colonoscopy and death from colorectal cancer. Ann Intern Med 2009;150:1–8.
9. Rex DK. Maximizing detection of adenomas and cancers during colonoscopy. Am J Gastroenterol 2006;101:2866–77.
10. Chen SC, Rex DK. Endoscopist can be more powerful than age and male gender in predicting adenoma detection at colonoscopy. Am J Gastroenterol 2007;102:856–61.
11. Lieberman DA, Weiss DG, Harford WV, et al. Five-year colon surveillance after screening colonoscopy. Gastroenterology 2007;133:1077–85.

12. Farrar WD, Sawhney MS, Nelson DB, et al. Colorectal cancers found after a complete colonoscopy. Clin Gastroenterol Hepatol 2004;4:1259–64.
13. van Rijn JC, Reitsma JB, Stoker J, et al. Polyp miss rate deter- mined by tandem colonoscopy: a systematic review. Am J Gastroenterol 2006;101:343–50.
14. Barclay RL, Vicari JJ, Doughty AS, et al. Colonoscopic withdrawal times and adenoma detection during screening colonoscopy. N Engl J Med 2006;355: 2533–41.
15. Barclay RL, Vicari JJ, Greenlaw RL. Effect of a time-dependent colonoscopic withdrawal protocol on adenoma detection during screening colonoscopy. Clin Gastroenterol Hepatol 2008;6:1091–8.
16. Sporea I, Popescu A, Vernic C, et al. How to improve the performances in diagnostic colonoscopy? J Gastrointestin Liver Dis 2007;16:363–7.
17. Radaelli F, Meucci G, Sgroi G, et al. Technical performance of colonoscopy: the key role of sedation/analgesia and other quality indicators. Am J Gastroenterol 2008;103:1122–30.
18. Sawhney MS, Cury MS, Neeman N, et al. Effect of institution-wide policy of colonoscopy withdrawal time > or = 7 minutes on polyp detection. Gastroenterology 2008;135:1892–8.
19. Shaukat A, Oancea Bond J, Curch TR, et al. Variation in detection of adenomas and polyps by colonoscopy and change over time with a performance improvement program. Clin Gastroenterol Hepatol 2009;7:1335–40.
20. Allen JI. Community colonoscopy: a gordian knot? Gastroenterology 2010;138: 27–30.
21. Morris SJ. The best value for our patients. AGA Perspectives 2010;6:4–6.
22. Schoen RE, Pinsky PF, Weissfeld JL, et al. Utilization of surveillance colonoscopy in community practice. Gastroenterology 2010;138:73–81.
23. Mysliwiec PA, Brown ML, Klabunde CN, et al. Are physicians doing too much colonoscopy? (A national survey of colorectal surveillance after polypectomy.) Ann Intern Med 2004;141:264–71.
24. Allen JI. A performance improvement program for community-based gastroenterology. Gastrointest Endosc Clin N Am 2008;18:753–71.
25. De Brantes F, Rosenthal MB, Painter M. building a bridge from fragmentation to accountability – the Prometheus payment model. N Engl J Med 2009;361:1033–6.
26. Fisher ES, McClellan MB, Bertko J, et al. Fostering accountable care: moving forward in Medicare. Health Aff 2009;28:w219–31.
27. Mandel KE. Aligning rewards with large-scale improvement. JAMA 2010;303: 663–4.

Index

Note: Page numbers of article titles are in **boldface** type.

A

Adenoma(s)
 conventional, management of, endoscopist–pathologist partnership in, 645–649
 detection of, colonoscopy in, efficacy of, 674
 invasive, management of, endoscopist–pathologist partnership in, 653–654
 sessile serrated, surveillance intervals for, endoscopist–pathologist partnership in,
  652–653
AERs. See Automated endoscope reprocessors (AERs).
American Society of Anesthesiologists (ASA), on colonoscopy reports, 686–687
Anesthesia/anesthetics, for colonoscopy, costs of, 759
Anticoagulation, in colonoscopy, 598
ASA. See American Society of Anesthesiologists (ASA).
Automated endoscope reprocessors (AERs), in reducing infection risk in endoscopy unit,
 609–610

B

Bowel preparation, for colonoscopy, complications of, 662–663

C

Cancer(s)
 colon
  missed, on colonoscopy, 597–598
  pathology of, current concepts of, 644–645
 colorectal. See Colorectal cancer.
Cardiovascular system, colonoscopy complications affecting, 660–662
Centers for Medicare and Medicaid Services (CMS), 723–724
Clinical Outcomes Research Initiative (CORI) experience, 729–730
CMS. See Centers for Medicare and Medicaid Services (CMS).
Colon, polyps of, pathology of, current concepts of, 644–645
Colon cancer
 missed, on colonoscopy, 597–598
 pathology of, current concepts of, 644–645
Colonoscopy
 assessment of
  advanced systems in, **699–716**
   EMIS, 704–713. See also Endoscopic Multimedia Information System (EMIS).
  future plans for, 713–715
 complications of, **659–671**
  bowel preparation–related, 662–663
  cardiovascular, 660–662
  described, 659

Gastrointest Endoscopy Clin N Am 20 (2010) 783–789
doi:10.1016/S1052-5157(10)00110-8
1052-5157/10/$ – see front matter © 2010 Elsevier Inc. All rights reserved.

United States Postal Service

Statement of Ownership, Management, and Circulation
(All Periodicals Publications Except Requester Publications)

1. Publication Title	2. Publication Number	3. Filing Date
Gastrointestinal Endoscopy Clinics of North America	0 1 2 - 6 0 0 3	9/15/10

4. Issue Frequency	5. Number of Issues Published Annually	6. Annual Subscription Price
Jan, Apr, Jul, Oct	4	$290.00

7. Complete Mailing Address of Known Office of Publication (Not printer) (Street, city, county, state, and ZIP+4®)

Elsevier Inc.
360 Park Avenue South
New York, NY 10010-1710

Contact Person
Stephen Bushing

Telephone (Include area code)
215-239-3688

8. Complete Mailing Address of Headquarters or General Business Office of Publisher (Not printer)

Elsevier Inc., 360 Park Avenue South, New York, NY 10010-1710

9. Full Names and Complete Mailing Addresses of Publisher, Editor, and Managing Editor (Do not leave blank)

Publisher (Name and complete mailing address)

Kim Murphy, Elsevier, Inc., 1600 John F. Kennedy Blvd. Suite 1800, Philadelphia, PA 19103-2899

Editor (Name and complete mailing address)

Kerry Holland, Elsevier, Inc., 1600 John F. Kennedy Blvd. Suite 1800, Philadelphia, PA 19103-2899

Managing Editor (Name and complete mailing address)

Catherine Bewick, Elsevier, Inc., 1600 John F. Kennedy Blvd. Suite 1800, Philadelphia, PA 19103-2899

10. Owner (Do not leave blank. If the publication is owned by a corporation, give the name and address of the corporation immediately followed by the names and addresses of all stockholders owning or holding 1 percent or more of the total amount of stock. If not owned by a corporation, give the names and addresses of the individual owners. If owned by a partnership or other unincorporated firm, give its name and address as well as those of each individual owner. If the publication is published by a nonprofit organization, give its name and address.)

Full Name	Complete Mailing Address
Wholly owned subsidiary of	4520 East-West Highway
Reed/Elsevier, US holdings	Bethesda, MD 20814

11. Known Bondholders, Mortgagees, and Other Security Holders Owning or Holding 1 Percent or More of Total Amount of Bonds, Mortgages, or Other Securities. If none, check box ☐ None

Full Name	Complete Mailing Address
N/A	

12. Tax Status (For completion by nonprofit organizations authorized to mail at nonprofit rates) (Check one)
The purpose, function, and nonprofit status of this organization and the exempt status for federal income tax purposes:
☐ Has Not Changed During Preceding 12 Months
☐ Has Changed During Preceding 12 Months (Publisher must submit explanation of change with this statement)

PS Form 3526, September 2007 (Page 1 of 3 (Instructions Page 3)) PSN 7530-01-000-9931 PRIVACY NOTICE: See our Privacy policy in www.usps.com

13. Publication Title	14. Issue Date for Circulation Data Below
Gastrointestinal Endoscopy Clinics of North America	July 2010

15. Extent and Nature of Circulation			Average No. Copies Each Issue During Preceding 12 Months	No. Copies of Single Issue Published Nearest to Filing Date
a. Total Number of Copies (Net press run)			975	900
b. Paid Circulation (By Mail and Outside the Mail)	(1)	Mailed Outside-County Paid Subscriptions Stated on PS Form 3541 (Include paid distribution above nominal rate, advertiser's proof copies, and exchange copies)	341	350
	(2)	Mailed In-County Paid Subscriptions Stated on PS Form 3541 (Include paid distribution above nominal rate, advertiser's proof copies, and exchange copies)		
	(3)	Paid Distribution Outside the Mails Including Sales Through Dealers and Carriers, Street Vendors, Counter Sales, and Other Paid Distribution Outside USPS®	164	165
	(4)	Paid Distribution by Other Classes Mailed Through the USPS (e.g. First-Class Mail®)		
c. Total Paid Distribution (Sum of 15b (1), (2), (3), and (4))		▶	505	515
d. Free or Nominal Rate Distribution (By Mail and Outside the Mail)	(1)	Free or Nominal Rate Outside-County Copies Included on PS Form 3541	85	83
	(2)	Free or Nominal Rate In-County Copies Included on PS Form 3541		
	(3)	Free or Nominal Rate Copies Mailed at Other Classes Through the USPS (e.g. First-Class Mail)		
	(4)	Free or Nominal Rate Distribution Outside the Mail (Carriers or other means)		
e. Total Free or Nominal Rate Distribution (Sum of 15d (1), (2), (3) and (4))		▶	85	83
f. Total Distribution (Sum of 15c and 15e)		▶	590	598
g. Copies not Distributed (See instructions to publishers #4 (page #3))		▶	385	302
h. Total (Sum of 15f and g)		▶	975	900
i. Percent Paid (15c divided by 15f times 100)			85.59%	86.12%

16. Publication of Statement of Ownership

☐ If the publication is a general publication, publication of this statement is required. Will be printed in the October 2010 issue of this publication.   ☐ Publication not required

17. Signature and Title of Editor, Publisher, Business Manager, or Owner

(signature)   Date

Stephen R. Bushing – Fulfillment/Inventory Specialist   September 15, 2010

I certify that all information furnished on this form is true and complete. I understand that anyone who furnishes false or misleading information on this form or who omits material or information requested on the form may be subject to criminal sanctions (including fines and imprisonment) and/or civil sanctions (including civil penalties).

PS Form 3526, September 2009 (Page 2 of 3)

Moving?

Make sure your subscription moves with you!

To notify us of your new address, find your **Clinics Account Number** (located on your mailing label above your name), and contact customer service at:

Email: journalscustomerservice-usa@elsevier.com

800-654-2452 (subscribers in the U.S. & Canada)
314-447-8871 (subscribers outside of the U.S. & Canada)

Fax number: 314-447-8029

Elsevier Health Sciences Division
Subscription Customer Service
3251 Riverport Lane
Maryland Heights, MO 63043

*To ensure uninterrupted delivery of your subscription, please notify us at least 4 weeks in advance of move.

Printed and bound by CPI Group (UK) Ltd, Croydon, CR0 4YY

03/10/2024

01040449-0001